Promoting
Family
Involvement
in **Long-Term
Care Settings**

Promoting
Family
Involvement
in **Long-Term**
Care Settings

A GUIDE TO PROGRAMS THAT WORK

edited by

Joseph E. Gaugler, Ph.D.

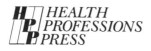
HEALTH
PROFESSIONS
PRESS

Baltimore • London • Sydney

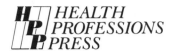

Health Professions Press, Inc.
Post Office Box 10624
Baltimore, Maryland 21285-0624

www.healthpropress.com

Typeset by International Graphic Services, Inc., Newtown, Pennsylvania.
Manufactured in the United States of America by
Versa Press, East Peoria, Illinois.

The photograph on the cover is used by permission of the individuals pictured.

Some of the case studies described in this book are based on the authors' actual experienxes. In these instances, names and identifying details have been changed to protect privacy. Other case studies are fictional accounts that do not represent the lives of specific individuals, and no implications should be inferred.

Library of Congress Cataloging-in-Publication Data
Promoting family involvement in long-term care settings : a guide to pro-
    grams that work / edited by Joseph E. Gaugler.
        p.   cm.
    Includes bibliographical references and index.
    ISBN-13: 978-1-932529-07-4
    ISBN-10: 1-932529-07-1
    1. Nursing homes—United States—Administration.   2. Long-term care
    facilities—United States—Administration.   3. Nursing homes—Patients—
    United States—Family relationships.   4. Long-term care facilities—
    Patients—United States—Family relationships.   5. Medical personnel-
    caregiver relationships—United States.   I. Gaugler, Joseph E.
    [DNLM: 1. Homes for the Aged.   2. Nursing Homes.   3. Caregivers—
    psychology.   4. Long-Term Care—methods—Aged.   5. Professional–Fam-
    ily Relations.   6. Professional–Patient Relations.   WT 27.1 P965 2005]
    RA997.P77 2005
    362.16—dc22   2005025131

British Library Cataloguing in Publication data are available from the British Library.

Contents

About the Editor

Joseph E. Gaugler, Ph.D., Assistant Professor, Center on Aging, Center for Gerontological Nursing, School of Nursing, The University of Minnesota, 5-160 Weaver-Densford Hall, 1331, 308 Harvard Street S.E., Minneapolis, MN 55455

Dr. Gaugler is currently Assistant Professor in the School of Nursing at The University of Minnesota. He is also a faculty member of The Center on Aging and Center for Gerontological Nursing at The University of Minnesota. Dr. Gaugler's research examines the sources and effectiveness of long-term care for older adults with chronic disabilities. As a developmental psychologist and Director of the Families and Long-Term Care Research Laboratory, Dr. Gaugler's specific interests include the longitudinal ramifications of family care for adults with disabilities, the effectiveness of community-based and psychosocial services for adults with chronic illness and their caregiving families, the social integration of residents in nursing homes and other emerging models of long-term care (e.g., assisted living, family care homes), and developmental methodology.

Dr. Gaugler currently serves on the editorial boards of *The Gerontologist* and *Psychology and Aging*. He was awarded the 2003 Springer Early Career Achievement Award in Adult Development and Aging Research from the American Psychological Association (Division 20: Adult Development and Aging).

Contributors

Keith A. Anderson, M.S.W.
Doctoral Candidate
Graduate Center for Gerontology
University of Kentucky
306 Wethington Health Sciences
  Building
900 South Limestone
Lexington, Kentucky 40536

Jennifer G. Basham, B.S.W.
Research Assistant
Department of Behavioral Science,
  College of Medicine
University of Kentucky
138 College of Medicine Office
  Building
Lexington, Kentucky 40536

Wayne A. Caron, Ph.D.
Senor Lecturer and Assistant
  Professor
Department of Family Social Science
University of Minnesota
290 McNeal Hall
1985 Buford Avenue
St. Paul, Minnesota 55108

Judith C. Drew, Ph.D., RN
Professor
The Joseph B. & Mary Alice
  Collerain Professorship
The University of Texas Medical
  Branch School of Nursing
301 University Boulevard
Route 1029
Galveston, Texas 77555

Kenneth Hepburn, Ph.D.
Professor and Associate Dean for
  Research
University of Minnesota
School of Nursing
308 Harvard Street, SE
Minneapolis, Minnesota 55455

Meridean L. Maas, Ph.D., RN
Emeritus Professor and Director
John A. Hartford Center of Geriatric
  Nursing Excellence
College of Nursing
University of Iowa
430 Nursing Building
Iowa City, Iowa 52246

Philip McCallion, Ph.D.
Center for Excellence in Aging
  Services
University at Albany
135 Western Avenue
Richardson Hall
Albany, New York 12222

Katherina A. Nikzad, B.A.
Research Fellow
Graduate Center for Gerontology
University of Kentucky
306 Health Sciences Building
900 South Limestone
Lexington, Kentucky 40536

Terry Peak, M.S.W, Ph.D.
Director
Social Work Program
Department of Sociology, Social
  Work & Anthropology
Utah State University
0730 Old Main Hill
Logan, Utah 84322

Karl A. Pillemer, Ph.D.
Professor
Human Development
Cornell University
G44 Martha Van Rensselaer Hall
Ithaca, New York 14853

David Reed, Ph.D.
Statistician
The University of Iowa College of
    Nursing
50 Newton Road
414 Nursing Building
Iowa City, Iowa 52242

Julie Robison, Ph.D.
Assistant Professor
Center on Aging, University of
    Connecticut Health Center
263 Farmington Avenue
Farmington, Connecticut
    06030-6147

**Janet K. Pringle Specht, Ph.D.,
    RN**
Associate Professor
University of Iowa College of
    Nursing
50 Newton Road
432 Nursing Building
Iowa City, Iowa 52242

Valerie E. Tolbert, Ph.D.
Post-doctoral Research Fellow
Department of Behavioral Science,
    College of Medicine
University of Kentucky
138 College of Medicine Office
    Building
Lexington, Kentucky 40536

Foreword

Despite recent efforts to transform nursing homes into friendlier, more homelike places, nursing homes continue to generate mostly negative images. Anticipating relocation to a nursing home often evokes fear and anxiety for both the older adult and his or her family members. We know that families do not end their caring, vigilance, or contact with their older relatives following a move into a nursing home. However, older adults generally fear that they will be abandoned and that they will be separated from the things that bring meaning to their lives, the things that are familiar and comfortable. At the same time families, regardless of their continued involvement, often feel they have abandoned their older, vulnerable relatives to the care of strangers.

For millions of nursing homes residents and their families, this is an urgent problem. Nursing home residents, like the rest of us, rely on important, continuing personal relationships to maintain meaningful lives. In research and personal accounts we are repeatedly reminded of how important both family and staff relationships are to nursing home residents. Most residents eagerly anticipate visits from family members, fill their rooms with pictures of family, and enjoy interacting with staff about what their families are doing.

The importance of relationships in general is underscored by the research on how residents evaluate care quality. This research tells us that the most important component of care quality is the quality of relationships between residents and staff. The great importance of these relationships is also reflected in residents' reluctance, even when they are distressed, to complain about the quality of care they are receiving.

Residents fear that complaints will result in reprimands to the caregiver they have become attached to or that the caregiver's feelings will be hurt. It is not surprising that frontline nursing staff members often describe their relationships with residents as being like family and the most rewarding aspect of the work. In fact, they often see themselves as standing in the place of family.

There is no question that it is quite comforting for both residents and family members when a resident is treated with affection and seen as having an important relationship with a staff member. While we can applaud the efforts of staff to see nursing home residents as family members and to nurture these relationships we might wonder, however, whether residents would be better served if their relationships

with family members were nurtured and supported following relocation to a nursing home. Nurturing relationships with families might
well require skillful assistance from staff committed to maintaining
important relationships in the residents' lives. It would also likely
require effective and positive relationships between family and staff.

What we know about relationships between family and staff, much
of which is described in this book, is that family–staff relationships are
frequently characterized by tension, misunderstandings, and unmet
expectations. This may discourage family visiting, may undermine relationships between family and residents, and can even prevent families
from advocating for their relatives, fearing retribution. Failure to
develop effective family–staff relationships will, at the very least, prevent staff from assisting families to maintain close relationships with
their elderly relatives.

The dynamics of these relationships are indeed complex. Important
questions remain unanswered and difficult problems remain unsolved,
creating an ideal opportunity for collaboration between researchers
and care providers. The nursing home industry has made significant
efforts to transform the lives of residents: improving the care, increasing
the choices they have over their daily lives, and focusing more on the
quality-of-life aspects of nursing home life. Generally known as culture
change initiatives, these programs have sprung up around the United
States and around the world. Curiously, none of these initiatives has
made resident–family relationships central features of its reforms.
Although included as an aspect of some, family–staff relationships have
not been pivotal in any of these programs. Considering the importance
of relationships, and the well-documented difficulty experienced in
family–staff relationships and resident–family relationships, this seems
an unfortunate oversight that has potentially serious consequences
for everyone.

These initiatives have provided us with some insights into programs
that have worked and those that have not. However, replication has
been largely unsuccessful since there is not often an adequate explanation for why something worked. Lack of insight into why something
works also makes sustainability difficult. We have seen this in many
promising initiatives, where good outcomes were achieved but replication was not successful. The absence of good data about program success
or failure and the absence of a theoretical basis for program development has hindered the development and ongoing support of these
novel and promising programs.

*Promoting Family Involvement in Long-Term Care Settings: A Guide to
Programs that Work* begins to address these oversights. It is an unusual

book in that it combines academic concerns about theoretical explanations and credible evidence with more practical interests in the details of program development, the emotions of the actors involved, and the practical implications of program implementation. One of the most intriguing consequences of this theoretical/practical blend is that it brings the research community closer to the practice world while demonstrating to the more practical-minded readers the usefulness of considering the more theoretical questions and the evidence for successful implementation. It is designed to demonstrate practical approaches to increasing family involvement in nursing home care, to embed those approaches (whenever possible) into a theoretical context, while also demanding evidence of the program's effectiveness. As might be expected, the descriptions of various programs raise many new questions that could generate enough research questions for several productive careers.

The promise of this book is that it creates the infrastructure for productive partnerships between researchers and care providers. Each chapter is written to provide rich detail about one specific focus on the problem with family involvement, the goal that program implementers are attempting to achieve, the challenges encountered when implementing the program, the effectiveness of the program in relation to the goals, and the insights gained along the way.

For those who are interested, the chapters collectively provide a comprehensive review of literature on family involvement in nursing home care. For those who are in the trenches, struggling to improve family–staff and family–resident relationships, the descriptions in these chapters will guide you through a range of possibilities while significantly pointing out the bumps in the road that are likely to be encountered. Possibly most important, the structure of the book, and of each chapter, demonstrates simultaneously the challenges of conducting applied research in nursing home settings (especially with families) and some promising strategies to deal with these challenges.

Barbara Bowers, Ph.D., RN, FAAN
Helen Denne Schulte Professor of Nursing
University of Wisconsin–Madison

Acknowledgments

I would like to thank all of the chapter contributors for their efforts in translating their important research into policy that can better the lives of older adults, their families, and those individuals who care for both.

I would also like to thank the staff at Health Professions Press—Mary Magnus, Amy Kopperude, Amy Perkins, and Stefanie Pawelczyk—for their tireless effort in promoting and formatting this volume so that it is as useful as possible.

Promoting
Family
Involvement
in **Long-Term**
Care Settings

Introduction

1

The Role of Families in Nursing Homes

JOSEPH E. GAUGLER

Although the myth prevails that families tend to abandon older adult relatives who live in nursing homes or similar settings, research since the 1970s has helped to debunk this perception (e.g., Bowers, 1988; Maas et al., 2000; Rowles & High, 1996; Smith & Bengtson, 1979; York & Calsyn, 1977; Zarit & Whitlatch, 1992). In contrast, family members appear to remain involved in various ways in the lives of residents in long-term care facilities, and in some instances this family involvement is linked to positive outcomes on the part of residents and even family members. This has led to several efforts to determine how family involvement is most effectively maximized and integrated in residential facilities to enhance resident quality of life, family well-being, and staff job satisfaction (e.g., Hepburn et al., 1997; Maas et al., 2000; Pillemer et al., 2003).

The purpose of this book and its subsequent chapters is to present several programs that have demonstrated potential for enhancing family involvement in nursing homes. In addition to providing readers with conceptual background and evaluation results, an ongoing emphasis

---

Available studies of family involvement in nursing homes were reviewed, and articles that were primarily anecdotal were excluded. The literature search was conducted on the MEDLINE, PsycINFO, CINAHL, and AgeLine databases using key terms such as "family involvement in long-term care," "families in nursing homes," "family" and "nursing homes," "visits" and "nursing homes," "family caregiving" and "nursing homes," "family care" and "nursing homes," and "informal care/help in nursing homes." A snowball strategy was used; the references of studies located in our initial database searches were examined to identify additional analyses of interest.

throughout each chapter is on the barriers to and challenges of implementing similar programs in a long-term care setting. In this respect, this book represents more than a simple summary of existing research; it is also a true guide for practitioners, families, and others to identify approaches that are best suited to their own particular residential environments and experiences.

This introductory chapter serves to ground and organize the subsequent chapters by providing an overview of what is known about family involvement in nursing homes. What does state-of-the-art research tell us about how family involvement occurs in nursing homes? What accounts for high or low levels of family involvement? How does family integration have an impact on important outcomes such as resident quality of life? This chapter then highlights some of the limitations of family involvement research and the need for ongoing work in this area, whether it is more descriptive or based on interventions such as those programs reviewed in this book.

DESCRIBING FAMILY INVOLVEMENT

Early studies of families and nursing homes tended to emphasize the potential isolation residents experienced. For example, researchers characterized the admission of an older adult to a nursing home as the "nadir" of life, or a time of intensified isolation and depression experienced by both family members and residents (Cath, 1972; Jones, 1972). Additional work on family involvement in long-term care viewed the family member as interfering, disruptive, and critical of professional policies, staff, and the overall facility environment (Bates, 1968; Blum, 1960). A special task force organized by Ralph Nader in 1970 designed to highlight the deficiencies of nursing home care found that 60% of residents in 10 nursing homes in West Virginia received visitors once a week, and the other 40% were visited once a month or less (Townsend, 1971). The findings indicated that many residents did not receive regular visitors, but the nonscientific nature of this inquiry makes it difficult to determine the reliability of the findings. This section synthesizes and critiques the findings of subsequent research describing family involvement.

Visiting

Various research efforts have attempted to determine how often family members visit relatives in residential long-term care settings (particularly nursing homes). Research throughout the 1970s sought to dispute the notion that families "dumped" their relatives in nursing homes to relinquish responsibility, leaving residents in isolation. For example, data collected from the 1973–1974 National Nursing Homes Surveys indicated that many nursing home residents received visitors; 61% of residents were visited at least once a week, whereas 25% were visited less than weekly. Only 11% of residents received no visitors. The majority of residents (50.3%) received visits from children (National Center for Health Statistics, 1977, 1979). Similar classic research suggested a similar frequency of nursing home visits (Gottesman, 1974; Spasoff et al., 1978).

Later work tended to focus on family visits more explicitly. Efforts that focused on both qualitative (or narrative/open-ended information) and empirical/numerical data suggested that the quality of family–resident relationships remained strong for many families and that visits tended to occur more than once a week (Smith & Bengtson, 1979; York & Calsyn, 1977). A considerable amount of research since the 1980s has reiterated these findings; families tend to visit residents in nursing homes at least once a week, if not more often. These findings remain similar, even for residents who have severe dementia (Bitzan & Kruzich, 1990; Hook, Sobal, & Oak, 1982; Monahan, 1995; Moss & Kurland, 1979; Tornatore & Grant, 2002).

Although the research cited previously tended to be cross-sectional ("one shot in time" research designs), other studies have examined family visits over time. Although cross-sectional studies tend to suggest that length of stay is negatively correlated to family visits (i.e., the longer the resident has been in the nursing home, the less often families visit), studies that actually examine family visits over time have found otherwise. Follow-up studies ranging from 2 weeks to 9 months to 2 years have found either stability in the number of nursing home visits or even increases (Aneshensel, Pearlin, Mullan, Zarit, & Whitlatch, 1995; Gaugler, Zarit, & Pearlin, 2003; Port et al., 2001; Ross, Rosenthal, & Dawson, 1997), and, in some instances, these visits tended to last from 2 to 4 hours on average.

The existing literature tends to support the notion that family members continue to remain involved in the lives of relatives following admission to a nursing home. Although the frequency and duration of visits vary somewhat, the data certainly seem to dispute the perception that families leave the residents in isolation. Several limitations are apparent in the existing literature, however. Most studies tend to analyze data from a single type of informant (e.g., residents, family members, staff) on family visits, and issues such as social desirability, recall error, and an overall lack of reliability in hour estimates may influence the accuracy of this information. Considering multiple sources (e.g., residents, family members, staff) when gathering data on degree of family visits would offer greater insight into how often family involvement actually occurs.

Types of Family Involvement

Although family members often provide the majority of care to relatives with disabilities while living in the community (e.g., Whitlatch & Noelker, 1996), an important change can take place when admission to a nursing home occurs. Some researchers have suggested that family care in nursing homes is based on the concept of "dual specialization" (Dobrof & Litwak, 1977; Litwak, 1985): Staff members tend to provide personal, "hands-on" care, whereas family members offer more emotional and psychological support to residents. However, Moss and Kurland (1979) found that most family members (72%) did a number of "special things for the resident that might not otherwise be done" (p. 274), such as grooming, cheering up the resident, or having conversations with the resident. Linsk, Miller, Pflaum, and Ortigara-Vick (1988) found that family members were involved in a similar range of activities, such as talking with the resident, holding hands or touching the resident, and helping the resident with grooming. Other research has emphasized that families continued to feel responsible for a wide range of tasks, including personal tasks (e.g., grooming, clipping fingernails), instrumental tasks (e.g., doing laundry, arranging for hair styling, shopping for the resident), and socioemotional tasks (e.g., writing letters, maintaining the resident's apartment, dealing with family guilt feelings), after nursing home admission (Bonder, Miller, & Linsk, 1991; Rubin & Shuttlesworth, 1983; Schwarz & Vogel, 1990; Shuttlesworth, Rubin, & Duffy, 1982). Families also felt responsible for new dimensions of assistance not originally provided while the relative was cared for at home, such as reporting abuse to authorities, promoting family understanding of nursing home policies, and initiating actions to ensure good staff–family relations. When family members and staff were asked who had primary responsibility for such tasks, a considerable amount of role ambiguity was apparent (i.e., staff felt that a particular task was the nursing home's responsibility, whereas family members felt that certain care tasks remained their responsibility), suggesting the potential difficulty of negotiating care responsibilities between family members and care staff.

Additional research on the types of activities family members engage in revealed similar results. Stephens, Kinney, and Ogrocki

(1991) found that a greater proportion of 60 in-home caregivers provided help with activities of daily living (ADL) when compared with 60 family caregivers whose relatives had been admitted to nursing homes. Studies on caregiving costs and time use for older adults with cognitive impairments and their family caregivers reported that family caregivers tended to relinquish intensive ADL care to nursing home staff but remained socially involved with residents and offered other types of help, such as supervision and monitoring of quality of care (Max, Webber, & Fox, 1995; Moss, Lawton, Kleban, & Duhamel, 1993; Rice et al., 1993). Although many studies suggest that families tend to relinquish care responsibilities to staff, longitudinal analyses tend to suggest that family members provide considerable personal care over time (Aneshensel et al., 1995; Penrod, Kane, & Kane, 2000).

Additional efforts have utilized more open-ended, narrative approaches when studying family involvement in nursing homes. Findings suggested that family members do not discuss care for relatives in residential care in terms of task allocation, but instead describe care by its purpose (Bowers, 1988; Duncan & Morgan, 1994; Hertzberg, Ekman, & Axelsson, 2001; Karner, Montgomery, Dobbs, & Wittmaier, 1998; Keefe & Fancey, 2000; Kolb, 2000; Rowles & High, 1996; Tickle & Hull, 1995; Tilse, 1997). Family members emphasized that their main goal when helping residents in nursing homes was to preserve the identity of the older relative. Family members suggested that maintaining a relative's identity is best accomplished through positive relationships with staff. For example, many family members served as a teaching resource to staff members so that aides and nurses would provide more personalized care to the relative in the nursing home.

There are several limitations to our current understanding of the types of family care delivered in nursing homes. First, it is unknown how family members perceive their role after a relative's admission. Most studies examine the hands-on care family members provide; more socioemotional types of help or family members' interactions with staff (e.g., monitoring or directing care) are generally not considered. A more diverse consideration of family involvement in nursing homes is needed to determine the comprehensive role of families following a relative's admission.

FACTORS THAT INFLUENCE FAMILY INVOLVEMENT

Several dimensions appear to be predictive of family involvement in nursing homes. For example, early research found that preadmission telephone contact, geographic proximity of family members, family members who visited alone, and residents with shorter lengths of stay were all variables associated with more extensive family visits (Hook et al., 1982; York & Calsyn, 1977). Additional early work by Gottesman (1974) reported that residents in nonprofit nursing homes with a low proportion of public pay residents had more visitors in the month prior to the survey. Other work suggested the importance of facility characteristics and policies in facilitating family integration in nursing homes; several studies have indicated that facilities most oriented to treating families as "clients" also promoted extensive family involvement (Friedemann, Montgomery, Maiberger, & Smith, 1997; Friedemann, Montgomery, Rice, & Farrell, 1999; Montgomery, 1982). However, the relationship between facility setting and family integration appears complex; when types of involvement such as hands-on care by family members were not promoted by the facility, this did not dissuade some families from continuing to provide this care.

Prospective research has also identified a wide array of factors associated with family involvement in nursing homes. A large-scale study of 1,441 nursing home residents by Port et al. (2001) reported that preadmission contact, contacts who were spouses or adult children, geographic proximity, less cognitive impairment of the relative, and Caucasian racial identity reliably predicted more frequent postadmission visits. An analysis of 185 caregivers of relatives with dementia prior to and following nursing home admission found that caregivers with less formal education, caregivers who provided at-home care for shorter periods of time, residents with a greater duration of stay in the nursing home, and residents with a lower frequency of behavior problems prior to admission were all indicators that appeared to account for more frequent family visits (Gaugler, Leitsch, Zarit, & Pearlin, 2000). A study by Max and associates (1995) also examined predictors of family care for individuals with cognitive impairments living in nursing homes: Residents who were younger, caregivers who were younger, nonspousal caregivers, caregivers who provided assistance for longer periods of time, caregivers who lived alone, residents who experienced fewer cognitive and functional impairments, and caregivers who were male were all variables significantly associated with the provision of family care following admission to a nursing home.

Predictors of family involvement have also been described in open-ended, qualitative studies. For example, Kelley, Swanson, Maas, and Tripp-Reimer (1999) examined reasons for visiting among family members of relatives admitted to special care units. Thirty randomly selected family members from a larger nursing home study (Maas et al., 2000) participated in a series of semistructured interviews. Content analyses revealed various predictors of family visits, such as family members' past interpersonal relationships with the resident, prior perceptions of nursing homes, and current social support from others. Reasons why family members visited included being faithful to the resident, being the "eyes and ears" of the resident, and being family. Kellett (1998, 1999) also examined family members' perceptions of caregiving in nursing homes via qualitative interview techniques. A series of semi-structured interviews with a small number of family members ($n = 14$) elicited several important themes in the process of family involvement. Motivation for and meaning of family involvement included sense of past family life, sense of a break from caregiving, sense of change in engaged involvement (i.e., shift from personal, hands-on care to more socioemotional support), sense of worth (i.e., possessing special knowl-edge), sense of concern, and sense of continuity. A major strength of these qualitative investigations is the recognition that family involve-ment is based in family relationships prior to admission; many quantita-tive studies have ignored family history when analyzing family involve-ment. As with other qualitative investigations of family involvement in long-term care, however, there is a glaring need to move beyond interviews with single family members and involve other important individuals in the nursing home experience.

FAMILY INVOLVEMENT AND RESIDENT OUTCOMES

A theme running through much of the available research is that family involvement is associated with positive outcomes on the part of resi-dents; however, few studies have examined the relationship between family involvement and resident psychosocial or functional outcomes. An early study by Noelker and Harel (1978) identified predictors of well-being and survival among 125 long-term care residents of 14 nursing homes. Regression models found that residents who had "met their desire for visitors" were more likely to report higher life satisfac-tion. In addition, Greene and Monahan (1982) determined whether family visits to nursing home residents affected psychosocial well-being. A random sample of 28 nursing homes and 298 residents within these facilities were included. Staff members were surveyed on a variety of dimensions, and subsequent empirical models found that a higher frequency of nursing home visits was associated with more positive psychosocial outcomes on the part of residents.

Subsequent research by Lewis, Kane, Cretin, and Clark (1985) identified determinants of resident discharge from nursing homes. Over a 2-year period, 563 residents from 24 nursing homes in Southern California were followed. Nursing notes provided information on family visits (coded as 0 = no; 1 = yes). Residents who received visitors were more likely to be discharged from a nursing home alive. Subsequent work by Penrod and colleagues (2000) attempted to determine whether informal care provided to residents during the 2 weeks following admission to a nursing home influenced discharge over a 6-week period. Caregivers providing the greatest informal assistance (i.e., more than 35 hours of care per week) were most likely to discharge their loved ones from a nursing home. Taken together, the findings suggest that informal care may potentially influence the quality of care that residents receive, possibly leading to discharge to the community.

Research by Kiely, Simon, Jones, and Morris (2000) examined the empirical relationship between nursing home resident social engagement and mortality over a 1,721-day interval. A total of 927 residents from a Boston, Massachusetts, nursing home were included. A 6-item scale of social engagement developed by Mor and colleagues (1995) was used. Residents with greater scores on the social engagement scale were less likely to die during the study. Although limited to one facility and to residents who could communicate, the long follow-up period and large sample provided additional results supporting the positive effects of social integration with important outcomes. Another large-scale study by Zimmerman, Gruber-Baldini, Hebel, Sloane, and Magaziner (2002) included 2,015 new admissions from 59 randomly sampled nursing homes in Maryland. In addition to a wide range of other factors, a greater percentage of facility visitors per every 100 beds was significantly associated with a slightly lower risk of infection and hospitalization for infection among nursing home residents.

DISCUSSION

Although prior research has adequately emphasized that family involvement exists in nursing homes, research efforts in other key areas (e.g., family involvement and resident outcomes) are relatively scant. For these reasons, the following discussion provides recommendations to refine the research of family involvement in residential long-term care. These recommendations are intended not only for descriptive research on family involvement in nursing homes but also for intervention efforts designed to facilitate and improve effective family involvement.

Existing research has tended to ignore the potentially diverse roles of family members following a relative's admission to a nursing home. Quantitative/numerical studies generally either analyze visits only or adopt task-based approaches based on ADL and instrumental activities of daily living (IADL) measures to determine range, and in some cases frequency, of family involvement. In contrast, qualitative research suggests that family members' roles move beyond the provision of personal and instrumental care to encompass assistance that is designed to preserve the identity and quality of life for residents in nursing homes (e.g., Bowers, 1988; Duncan & Morgan, 1994; Kelley et al., 1999; Rowles & High, 1996). Quantitative research that extends traditional ADL and IADL assessments to consider more socioemotional forms of help is needed to effectively capture family roles in nursing homes.

The literature also tends to assume that increased family involvement is positive and leads to quality of life and quality of care for residents. Relative to other research on family involvement, few studies exist that directly test this assertion. Prior work suggests that family involvement and increased social engagement lead to positive psychosocial outcomes (Greene & Monahan, 1982; Noelker & Harel, 1978); discharge to the community (Lewis et al., 1985; Penrod et al., 2000); and decreased mortality, infection, and hospitalization on the part of residents (Kiely et al., 2000; Zimmerman et al., 2002). Most of these studies solely examine family visits or ADL/IADL care provided and do not ascertain how other dimensions of family involvement (e.g., socioemotional support, advocacy) may affect residents. Given the multidimensional nature of family involvement and quality of life (e.g., Kane, 2001), future research must direct greater attention to the potentially complex associations between family involvement and various domains of resident outcomes.

Most analyses of family involvement utilize cross-sectional designs (i.e., residents or other individuals are assessed at only one point in time). Unfortunately, these designs represent a static method that may not accurately reflect change in family involvement over time. For example, cross-sectional findings often suggest that greater resident length of stay is associated with fewer family visits; however, prospective longitudinal research has found that many families continue to remain involved in the lives of residents in long-term care facilities (e.g., Aneshensel et al., 1995; Gaugler, Zarit, & Pearlin, 2003; Spasoff et al., 1978). Additional prospective research that includes larger, more representative samples and examines types of involvement in addition to frequency of visits will significantly add to our understanding of how family involvement shifts and changes over time.

Few studies examine family involvement among ethnically or racially diverse residents (for an exception, see Kolb, 2000). As in community caregiving (e.g., Dilworth-Anderson, 2001), family involvement within diverse ethnic or racial contexts may operate in a qualitatively different manner when compared with that for Caucasian residents. Examination of the process of family care and integration in these situations will offer a more representative picture of the transition to residential care for all family members of residents in nursing homes.

An important methodological challenge in residential long-term care research is attrition in resident, family, or staff samples. Death or failure to follow up in resident, family or staff samples can bias results in an empirical analysis; often those participants who remain in long-term studies are also among the most healthy and highest functioning nursing home residents. Stark, Kane, Kane, and Finch (1995) recommended several conservative approaches that can be included to address the effects of attrition bias in long-term care samples. For example, designs that include both those residents who remain in the study over time and those who exit (a resident's death is the main reason for exiting a nursing home; see Gaugler & Kane, 2001) can be utilized. Residents who die are assigned the lowest values on measures of importance, such as functional status, family involvement, and psychosocial well-being. Although this approach is conservative, it can potentially address attrition bias. Berk (1983), Heckman (1979), and Miller and Wright (1995) recommended several empirical approaches that can also be incorporated to counteract attrition bias in longitudinal evaluations (e.g., the Heckman two-stage approach; see Heckman, 1979). The Heckman adjustment can model the "decision" to leave a longitudinal evaluation and then use information about each person's likelihood of exiting the study (i.e., the Mills ratio) to correct for selective attrition bias.

An additional limitation in family involvement research is the inordinate focus on "primary" family members. The primary family member is the one caregiver who is most involved in the life of a resident following admission to a nursing home (Maas et al., 2000). There is usually one "primary" caregiver who provides the majority of help to older adults living in the community (Aneshensel et al., 1995; Cantor, 1983). However, other studies have emphasized that multiple family members can provide assistance to older people with impairments, illustrating the potential complexity of family caregiving (Dilworth-Anderson, 2001; Gaugler et al., 2000; Schoenberg, Amey, Stoller, & Muldoon, 2003; Tennstedt, McKinlay, & Sullivan, 1989). The dynamics of family structure, in terms of number of involved family members, their roles in involvement, and their interactions with facility staff, must be taken into account in both qualitative and quantitative efforts. Recognizing the multiple configurations of families may help to refine and facilitate staff–family care plans and relationships, and in some cases could prove integral to the successful involvement of not only a primary family member but also the entire family.

In contrast, some residents in a variety of long-term care settings have no family members at all, which complicates the interpretation of the findings in prior family involvement research. For example, findings suggest that family members who live closer to residents are more likely to visit when compared with family members who do not. However, these results often do not take into account those residents without family members, which adds considerable complexity to the role and potential influence of family involvement in residential long-term care. To date, it remains unknown how the lack of family members among older adults in residential long-term care affects key outcomes. Future research that recognizes and includes residents without family members or other social supports would add considerably to the family involvement literature and provide key information on how external social support influences older adults in residential long-term care.

Descriptive studies on family involvement following admission help provide initial information on families' roles and integration in nursing homes, but the existing research tends to be atheoretical. Better conceptual models are needed to determine the antecedents and effects of family involvement in residential long-term care. Such models would be useful both in guiding descriptive efforts and in developing interventions with the goal of facilitating family involvement. For example, Figure 1.1 illustrates a potential model of family involvement in residential long-term care that captures elements of family caregiving prior to admission (i.e., the stress process; see Aneshensel et al., 1995) as well as descriptive findings on the types and ramifications of family involvement. Specifically, the stress process model takes a multidimensional and comprehensive approach in describing how caregiving can become problematic before admission and highlights various precursors and outcomes, including the sociodemographic context of care, emotional and psychological reactions to care demands, and psychosocial resources that can affect negative outcomes related to stress. In addition to incorporating elements of the stress process, the conceptual model in Figure 1.1 considers the results of prior research in documenting the potential types of involvement among multiple family members in residential long-term care, their precursors, and potential outcomes

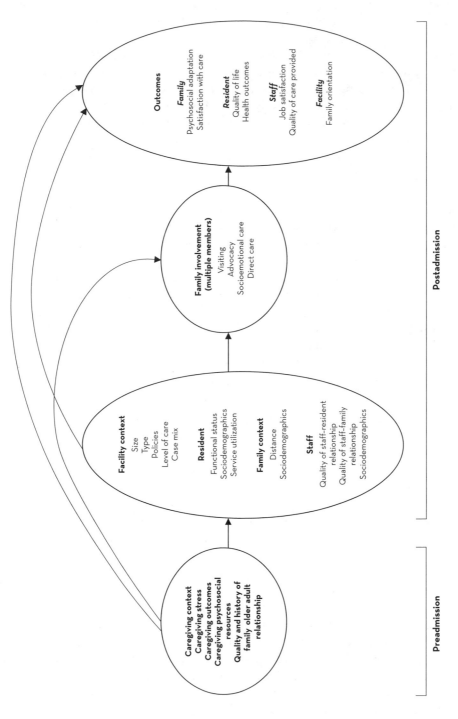

Figure 1.1. Conceptual model of family involvement in residential long-term care. (From Gaugler, J.E. [2005]. Family involvement in residential long-term care: A synthesis and critical review. *Aging and Mental Health*, 9, 115; reprinted by permission of Taylor & Francis, http://www.tandf.co.uk.)

among an array of stakeholders. An important component of the model is its emphasis on time; family–resident relationships have their genesis in lives prior to admission (Kelley et al., 1999).

A final recommendation, and one aimed at practitioners themselves, is the need for research participation, particularly in studies that attempt to evaluate novel programs designed to enhance family involvement. Although it is a growing area of research, there is little empirical evidence on how family involvement actually affects nursing home residents or what strategies are most effective in incorporating families into facility life. Understanding how families contribute to resident, staff, and facility outcomes via quality research can provide important insights to providers who are actively involved in quality-of-care and quality-of-life improvement efforts.

CONCLUSION

Early research on family involvement in nursing homes attempted to challenge the belief that families leave residents to die in isolation in nursing homes. As the existing research suggests, families often continue to visit and provide help to relatives in residential long-term care settings. The reasons why family members remain involved in the lives of relatives following admission to a nursing home are diverse; various facility-, resident-, and family-level variables all appear to predict family involvement. Some work has also linked family involvement to important resident outcomes, although the number of studies in this area is small. Although research on family involvement has advanced since the 1970s, prospective longitudinal studies, a consideration of the complex dynamics of family structure, and incorporation of pre- and postadmission conceptual models will advance the state of the art. These refinements will assist researchers, practitioners, and policy makers in adapting the nursing home environment into one that encourages appropriate family involvement and leads to more positive outcomes on the part of family members, residents, and staff.

REFERENCES

Aneshensel, C.S., Pearlin, L.I., Mullan, J.T., Zarit, S.H., & Whitlatch, C.J. (1995). *Profiles in caregiving: The unexpected career.* San Diego: Academic Press.
Bates, R.C. (1968). *The fine art of understanding patients.* Oradell, NJ: Medical Economics Book Division.

Berk, R.A. (1983). An introduction to sample selection bias in sociological data. *American Sociological Review, 48,* 386–398.

Bitzan, J.E., & Kruzich, J.M. (1990). Interpersonal relationships of nursing home residents. *The Gerontologist, 30,* 385–390.

Blum, R.H. (1960). *Management of the doctor–patient relationship.* New York: McGraw-Hill.

Bonder, B.R., Miller, B., & Linsk, N. (1991). Who should do what? Staff and family responsibilities for persons with Alzheimer's disease in nursing homes. *Clinical Gerontologist, 10,* 80–84.

Bowers, B.J. (1988). Family perceptions of care in a nursing home. *The Gerontologist, 28,* 361–368.

Cantor, M.H. (1983). Strain among caregivers: A study of experience in the United States. *The Gerontologist, 23,* 597–604.

Cath, S.H. (1972). The institutionalization of a parent: A nadir of life. *Journal of Geriatric Psychiatry, 5,* 25–46.

Dilworth-Anderson, P. (2001). Family issues and the care of persons with Alzheimer's disease. *Aging & Mental Health, 5,* S49–S51.

Dobrof, R.D., & Litwak, E. (1977). *Maintenance of family ties of long-term care patients.* Bethesda, MD: National Institute of Mental Health.

Duncan, M.T., & Morgan, D.L. (1994). Sharing the caring: Family caregivers' views of their relationships with nursing home staff. *The Gerontologist, 34*(2), 235–244.

Friedemann, M.L., Montgomery, R.J., Maiberger, B., & Smith, A.A. (1997). Family involvement in the nursing home: Family-oriented practices and staff–family relationships. *Research in Nursing and Health, 20,* 527–537.

Friedemann, M.L., Montgomery, R.J., Rice, C., & Farrell, L. (1999). Family involvement in the nursing home. *Western Journal of Nursing Research, 21,* 549–567.

Gaugler, J.E. (2005). Family involvement in residential long-term care: A synthesis and critical review. *Aging and Mental Health, 9,* 105–118.

Gaugler, J.E., & Kane, R.A. (2001). Informal help in the assisted living setting: A one-year analysis. *Family Relations, 50,* 335–347.

Gaugler, J.E., Leitsch, S.A., Zarit, S.H., & Pearlin, L.I. (2000). Caregiver involvement following institutionalization: Effects of pre-placement stress. *Research on Aging, 22,* 337–359.

Gaugler, J.E., Zarit, S.H., & Pearlin, L.I. (2003). Family involvement following institutionalization: Modeling nursing home visits over time. *International Journal of Aging and Human Development, 57,* 91–117.

Gottesman, L.E. (1974). Nursing home performance as related to resident traits, ownership, size, and source of payment. *American Journal of Public Health, 64,* 269–276.

Greene, V., & Monahan, D. (1982). The impact of visitation on patient well-being in nursing homes. *The Gerontologist, 22,* 418–423.

Heckman, J.J. (1979). Sample selection bias as specification error. *Econometrica, 47,* 153–161.

Hepburn, K.W., Caron, W., Luptak, M., Ostwald, S., Grant, L., & Keenan, J.M. (1997). The Families Stories Workshop: Stories for those who cannot remember. *The Gerontologist, 37,* 827–832.

Hertzberg, A., Ekman, S.L., & Axelsson, K. (2001). Staff activities and behaviour are the source of many feelings: Relatives' interactions and relationships with staff in nursing homes. *Journal of Clinical Nursing, 10,* 380–388.

Hook, W.F., Sobal, J., & Oak, J.C. (1982). Frequency of visitation in nursing homes: Patterns of contact across the boundaries of total institutions. *The Gerontologist, 22,* 424–428.

Jones, D.C. (1972). Social isolation, interaction, and conflict in two nursing homes. *The Gerontologist, 12,* 230–234.

Kane, R.A. (2001). Long-term care and a good quality of life: Bringing them closer together. *The Gerontologist, 41,* 293–304.

Karner, T.X., Montgomery, R.J.V., Dobbs, D., & Wittmaier, C. (1998, February). Increasing staff satisfaction: The impact of SCUs and family involvement. *Journal of Gerontological Nursing, 24,* 39–44.

Keefe, J., & Fancey, P. (2000). The care continues: Responsibility for elderly relatives before and after admission to a long term care facility. *Family Relations, 49,* 235–243.

Kellett, U.M. (1998). Meaning-making for family carers in nursing homes. *International Journal of Nursing Practice, 4,* 113–119.

Kellett, U.M. (1999). Transition in care: Family carers' experience of nursing home placement. *Journal of Advanced Nursing, 29,* 1474–1481.

Kelley, L.S., Swanson, E., Maas, M.L., & Tripp-Reimer, T. (1999, February). Family visitation on special care units. *Journal of Gerontological Nursing, 25,* 14–21.

Kiely, D.K., Simon, S.E., Jones, R.N., & Morris, J.N. (2000). The protective effect of social engagement on mortality in long-term care. *Journal of the American Geriatrics Society, 48,* 1367–1372.

Kolb, P.J. (2000). Continuing to care: Black and Latina daughters' assistance to their mothers in nursing homes. *Affilia: Journal of Women and Social Work, 15,* 502–525.

Lewis, M.A., Kane, R.L., Cretin, S., & Clark, V. (1985). The immediate and subsequent outcomes of nursing home care. *American Journal of Public Health, 75,* 758–762.

Linsk, N.L., Miller, B., Pflaum, R., & Ortigara-Vick, A. (1988). Families, Alzheimer's disease, and nursing homes. *Journal of Applied Gerontology, 7*(3), 331–349.

Litwak, E. (1985). *Helping the elderly: The complementary roles of informal networks and formal systems.* New York: Guilford Press.

Maas, M.L., Swanson, E., Buckwalter, K.C., Specht, J.P., Tripp-Reimer, T., Lenth, R., et al. (2000). *Final report: Nursing interventions for Alzheimer's: Family role trials* (RO1NR01689). Rockville, MD: National Institutes of Health.

Max, W., Webber, P., & Fox, P. (1995). Alzheimer's disease: The unpaid burden of caring. *Journal of Aging and Health, 7,* 179–199.

Miller, R.B., & Wright, D.W. (1995). Detecting and correcting attrition bias in longitudinal family research. *Journal of Marriage and the Family, 57,* 921–929.

Monahan, D.J. (1995). Informal caregivers of institutionalized dementia residents: Predictors of burden. *Journal of Gerontological Social Work, 23,* 65–82.

Montgomery, R.J.V. (1982). Impact of institutional care policies on family visitation. *The Gerontologist, 22,* 54–58.

Mor, V., Branco, K., Fleishman, J., Hawes, C., Phillips, C., Morris, J., et al. (1995). The structure of social engagement among nursing home residents. *Journals of Gerontology. Series B, Psychological Sciences and Social Sciences, 50,* P1–P8.

Moss, M.S., & Kurland, P. (1979). Family visiting with institutionalized mentally impaired aged. *Journal of Gerontological Social Work, 1,* 271–278.

Moss, M.S., Lawton, M.P., Kleban, M.H., & Duhamel, L. (1993). Time use of caregivers of impaired elderly before and after institutionalization. *Journal of Gerontology, 48,* S102–S111.

National Center for Health Statistics. (1977). Characteristics, social contacts, and activities of nursing home residents, United States, 1973–1974. *Vital and Health Statistics. Series 13: Data from the National Health Survey, No. 27.* DHEW Publication No. (HRA) 77-1778. Washington, DC: U.S. Department of Health, Education and Welfare.

National Center for Health Statistics. (1979). The national nursing home survey: 1977 summary for the United States. *Vital and Health Statistics. Series 13: Data from the National Health Survey, No. 43.* DHEW Publication (PHS) 79-1794. Washington, DC: U.S. Department of Health, Education and Welfare.

Noelker, L., & Harel, Z. (1978). Predictors of well-being and survival among institutionalized aged. *The Gerontologist, 18,* 562–567.

Penrod, J.D., Kane, R.A., & Kane, R.L. (2000). Effects of post-hospital informal care on nursing home discharge. *Research on Aging, 22,* 66–82.

Pillemer, K., Suitor, J.J., Henderson, C.R., Meador, R., Schultz, L., Robison, J., & Hegeman, C. (2003). A cooperative communication intervention for nursing home staff and family members of residents. *The Gerontologist, 43*(Special Issue II), 96–106.

Port, C.L., Gruber-Baldini, A.L., Burton, L., Baumgarten, M., Hebel, J.R., Zimmerman, S.I., et al. (2001). Resident contact with family and friends following nursing home admission. *The Gerontologist, 41,* 589–596.

Rice, D.P., Fox, P.J., Max, W., Webber, P.A., Lindeman, D.A., Hauck, W.W., et al. (1993). The economic burden of Alzheimer's disease care. *Health Affairs, 12,* 164–176.

Ross, M.M., Rosenthal, C., & Dawson, P. (1997). Spousal caregiving in the institutional setting: Visiting. *Journal of Clinical Nursing, 6,* 473–483.

Rowles, G.D., & High, D.M. (1996). Individualized care: Family roles in nursing home decision-making. *Journal of Gerontological Nursing, 22*(3), 20–25.

Rubin, A., & Shuttlesworth, G.E. (1983). Engaging families as support resources in nursing home care: Ambiguity in the subdivision of tasks. *The Gerontologist, 23,* 632–636.

Schoenberg, N.E., Amey, C.H., Stoller, E.P., & Muldoon, S.B. (2003). Lay referral patterns involved in cardiac treatment seeking among middle-aged and older adults. *The Gerontologist, 43,* 493–502.

Schwarz, A.N., & Vogel, M.E. (1990). Nursing home staff and residents' families role expectations. *The Gerontologist, 30,* 169–183.

Shuttlesworth, G.E., Rubin, A., & Duffy, M. (1982). Families versus institutions: Incongruent role expectations in the nursing home. *The Gerontologist, 22,* 200–208.

Smith, K.F., & Bengtson, V.L. (1979). Positive consequences of institutionalization: Solidarity between elderly patients and their middle-aged children. *The
Gerontologist, 19,* 438–447.

Spasoff, R.A., Kraus, A.S., Beattie, E.J., Holden, D.E.W., Lawson, J.S., Roden-
burg, M., et al. (1978). A longitudinal study of elderly residents in long-stay
institutions. *The Gerontologist, 18,* 281–292.

Stark, A.J., Kane, R.L., Kane, R.A., & Finch, M. (1995). Effect on physical
functioning of care in adult foster homes and nursing homes. *The Gerontologist,
35,* 648–655.

Stephens, M.A.P., Kinney, J.M., & Ogrocki, P.K. (1991). Stressors and well-
being among caregivers to older adults with dementia: The in-home versus
nursing home experience. *The Gerontologist, 31,* 217–223.

Tennstedt, S.L., McKinlay, J.B., & Sullivan, L.M. (1989) Informal care for frail
elders: The role of secondary caregivers. *The Gerontologist, 29,* 677–683.

Tickle, E.H., & Hull, K.V. (1995). Family members' roles in long-term care.
MEDSURG Nursing, 4, 300–304.

Tilse, C. (1997). She wouldn't dump me: The purpose and meaning of visiting
a spouse in residential care. *Journal of Family Studies, 3,* 196–208.

Tornatore, J.B., & Grant, L.A. (2002). Burden among family caregivers of
persons with Alzheimer's disease in nursing homes. *The Gerontologist, 42,* 497–
506.

Townsend, C. (1971). *Old age: The last segregation.* New York: Grossman Publish-
ers.

Whitlatch, C.J., & Noelker, L. (1996). Caregiving and caring. In A. Svanborg,
E.J. Masoro, K.W. Schaie, J.E. Birren, V.W. Marshall, & T.R. Cole (Eds.),
Encyclopedia of gerontology (Vol. 1, pp. 253–268). San Diego: Academic
Press.

York, J.L., & Calsyn, R.J. (1977). Family involvement in nursing homes. *The
Gerontologist, 17,* 500–505.

Zarit, S.H., & Whitlatch, C.J. (1992). Institutional placement: Phases of transition. *The Gerontologist, 32,* 665–672.

Zimmerman, S., Gruber-Baldini, A.L., Hebel, R., Sloane, P.D., & Magaziner, J.
(2002). Nursing home facility risk factors for infection and hospitalization:
Importance of registered nurse turnover, administration, and social factors.
Journal of the American Geriatrics Society, 50, 1987–1995.

RESOURCES

Dr. Gaugler is Assistant Professor in the Center on Aging and Center
for Gerontological Nursing in the University of Minnesota School of
Nursing. He has conducted a number of studies related to family caregiving and admission to long-term care facilities. A list of his publica-
tions is presented in this section; for more information about reprints
or the content of these studies, please contact

Joseph E. Gaugler, Ph.D.
Assistant Professor
School of Nursing
The University of Minnesota
6-150 Weaver-Densford Hall, 1331
308 Harvard Street S.E.
Minneapolis, MN 55455
E-mail: gaug0015@umn.edu
Phone: 612-626-2485
Fax: 612-626-2359

Publications/Reports

Gaugler, J.E. (2005). Family involvement in residential long-term care: A synthesis and critical review. *Aging & Mental Health, 9,* 105–118.

Gaugler, J.E., Anderson, K.A., & Leach, C.R. (2003). Predictors of family involvement in residential long-term care. *Journal of Gerontological Social Work, 42,* 3–26.

Gaugler, J.E., Anderson, K.A., Zarit, S.H., & Pearlin, L.I. (2004). Family involvement in the nursing home: Effects on stress and well-being. *Aging and Mental Health, 8,* 65–75.

Gaugler, J.E., Edwards, A.B., Femia, E.E., Zarit, S.H., Stephens, M.A.P., Townsend, A., et al. (2000). Predictors of institutionalization of cognitively impaired elders: Family help and the timing of placement. *Journals of Gerontology. Series B, Psychological Sciences and Social Sciences, 55,* P247–P255.

Gaugler, J.E., & Holmes, H.H. (2003). Families' experiences of nursing home placement: Adaptation and intervention. *The Clinical Psychologist, 7,* 32–43.

Gaugler, J.E., & Kane, R.A. (2001). Informal help in the assisted living setting: A one-year analysis. *Family Relations, 50,* 335–347.

Gaugler, J.E., Kane, R.L., Kane, R.A., Clay, T., & Newcomer, R. (2003). Predicting institutionalization of cognitively impaired older people: Utilizing dynamic predictors of change. *The Gerontologist, 43,* 219–229.

Gaugler, J.E., Kane, R.L., Kane, R.A., Clay, T., & Newcomer, R. (2005). The effects of duration of caregiving on institutionalization. *The Gerontologist, 45,* 78–89.

Gaugler, J.E., Kane, R.L., Kane, R.A., & Newcomer, R.C. (2005). Early community-based service utilization and its effects on institutionalization in dementia caregiving. *The Gerontologist, 45,* 78–89.

Gaugler, J.E., Leach, C.R., & Anderson, K.A. (2004). Correlates of resident psychosocial status in long-term care. *International Journal of Geriatric Psychiatry, 19,* 773–780.

Gaugler, J.E., Leach, C.R., Clay, T., & Newcomer, R. (2004). Predictors of nursing home placement in African-Americans with dementia. *Journal of the American Geriatrics Society, 52,* 445–452.

Gaugler, J.E., Leitsch, S.A., Zarit, S.H., & Pearlin, L.I. (2000). Caregiver involvement following institutionalization: Effects of preplacement stress. *Research on Aging, 22,* 337–359.

Gaugler, J.E., Pearlin, L.I., Leitsch, S.A., & Davey, A. (2001). Relinquishing in-home dementia care: Difficulties and perceived helpfulness during the nursing home transition. *American Journal of Alzheimer's Disease, 16,* 32–42.

Gaugler, J.E., Zarit, S.H., & Pearlin, L.I. (1999). Caregiving and institutionalization: Perceptions of family conflict and socioemotional support. *International Journal of Aging and Human Development, 49,* 15–38.

Gaugler, J.E., Zarit, S.H., & Pearlin, L.I. (2003). Family involvement following institutionalization: Modeling nursing home visits over time. *International Journal of Aging and Human Development, 57,* 91–117.

Manuscripts in Press

Anderson, K.A., Jui-Chang, J., Pearlin, L.I., Zarit, S.H., & Gaugler, J.E. (in press). Social class and the subjective adaptation of caregivers to institutionalization. *Journal of Social Work in Long-Term Care.*

Gaugler, J.E. (in press). Family involvement and resident psychosocial status in long-term care. *Clinical Gerontologist.*

Gaugler, J.E., Anderson, K.A., & Holmes, H.H. (2005). Family-based intervention in residential long-term care. *Marriage and Family Review, 37,* 45–62.

Gaugler, J.E., & Holmes, H.H. (in press). Determinants of staff attitudes toward family members in residential long-term care. *Journal of Gerontological Nursing.*

Manuscript Submitted for Publication

Gaugler, J.E., Kane, R.L., Kane, R.A., & Newcomer, R. (2005). Predictors of institutionalization in Latinos with dementia: A cross-cultural analysis. Manuscript submitted for publication.

Report

Gaugler, J.E., Anderson, K.A., & Leach, C.R. (2003). *Family involvement and quality of life in residential long-term care: Final report* (RO3 AG20786). Lexington: Department of Behavioral Science, The University of Kentucky.

I

Building and Refining
Existing Strategies

2

Family Councils in Residential Long-Term Care

KEITH A. ANDERSON

As past research has emphasized, family members continue to play active and important roles in the lives of their relatives following place-ment into residential long-term care (e.g., Aneshensel, Pearlin, Mullan, Zarit, & Whitlatch, 1995; Hook, Sobal, & Oak, 1982; Smith & Bengtson, 1979; York & Calsyn, 1977). The wide range of physical, social, and emotional supports provided by family members serves a number of purposes, including maintaining emotional and social bonds, aug-menting the care provided by the institution, monitoring the resident and the staff, and sustaining the roles that family members had fulfilled prior to admission. Active family involvement (e.g., visits, assistance with care) has been associated with several positive outcomes, such as feelings of satisfaction and usefulness in caregivers and an enhanced ability to individualize care (Ross, Rosenthal, & Dawson, 1997; Rowles & High, 1996; Tornatore & Grant, 2004). Family members may also be involved on a more formal, institutional level by serving on boards and councils that contribute to program and policy development within facilities. Family councils are groups that enable families to have input into the care that their relatives receive from nursing homes. This chapter discusses and reviews the functions, structure, philosophical foundations, and past research on family councils in long-term care facilities. In addition, it presents a best practice approach for establishing and maintaining an effective family council.

PURPOSES AND FUNCTIONS OF FAMILY COUNCILS

As a result of growing concern regarding the quality of residential long-term care, the Federal Nursing Home Reform Act (part of the Omnibus Budget Reconciliation Act of 1987 [PL 100-203], or OBRA 1987) was signed into law. Among a plethora of other actions aimed at improving the industry, OBRA 1987 formally mandated the right of family members to form family councils in long-term care institutions that receive Medicare and Medicaid funding. In addition, OBRA 1987 outlined the responsibilities of long-term care institutions to facilitate the establishment and maintenance of such groups. With regard to family councils, the law specifically delineated the following (§ 483.15[c]):

- A resident's family has the right to meet in the facility with the families of other residents.

- The facility must provide a private space for family council meetings.

- Staff or visitors may attend meetings at the group's invitation.

- The facility must provide a designated staff member responsible for providing assistance and responding to written requests that result from group meetings.

- The facility must listen to the views and act on the grievances and recommendations of residents and families concerning proposed policy and operational decisions affecting resident care and life at the facility.

   Based on these tenets, family councils are generally defined as "organized, self-led, self-determining, democratic group(s) composed of family members and friends of residents of long-term care facilities" (Bailey & Poole, 2004, p. 1). Family councils commonly consist of 5–10 family members and a staff liaison. The latter generally assists or "moderates" the group but is not considered an actual member. Family councils typically meet on a monthly basis in the facility in an area provided by the institution. Although staff members (e.g., social workers) occasionally serve as co-leaders of family council meetings, the groups are generally led by a family member chosen by the other council members. The findings, concerns, and suggestions that result from meetings are ideally forwarded to a designated staff member or to the facility administrator. Family councils may also relay their concerns to the long-term care ombudsman.

The specific goals and agendas of family councils tend to vary by composition and institution. Nevertheless, the general purposes of the groups are threefold: 1) to improve the quality of life and quality of care for the residents of long-term care institutions, 2) to give family members and friends a formal voice in the decision making of facilities, and 3) to facilitate communication between family members and facility administration. Stemming from these three general goals, family councils may focus on several specific purposes, including the following (Hart, Rehwaldt, & Clark, 1994):

- *Support:* providing mutual support and sharing in the experience of having a family member in long-term care. This includes welcoming new family members and helping family members adjust to the many changes introduced by the institutional environment.

- *Education:* providing education to family members regarding the functioning of the institution and the rights and responsibilities of residents, family members, and staff members. Sharing "insider knowledge" of the realities of institutional life is an important component of the educational function of family councils.

- *Advocacy:* addressing the concerns and problems encountered by residents and family members in the facility. This includes interfacing with the institution through board meetings and committees and working through local, state, and federal agencies to address problems and improve institutional care.

- *Communication:* providing family members with a voice in the institution and facilitating communication between family members, residents, and the institution. Inadequate and ineffective communication between families and staff is frequently listed as a major concern in long-term care institutions (Hertzberg & Ekman, 1996; Pillemer, 1996). Family councils allow both direct-care staff and administrators to hear an aggregate voice from family members, thereby enhancing communication and expediting the problem-solving process.

- *Services and activities:* providing input on the services and activities that take place in the institution. This function of the family council is intended to be a constructive, cooperative effort among families, residents, and staff to organize and direct activities and services that add to the lives of all of the involved parties.

PHILOSOPHICAL
FOUNDATIONS OF FAMILY COUNCILS

Family councils in long-term care facilities were established to improve
the quality of care of residents and to allow family members and friends
to have a formal voice in the institution. Three philosophical concepts
support these goals: empowerment, advocacy, and support. Understanding these terms offers insight into the mechanics of family councils
and the theoretical foundations on which they stand.

Empowerment

Empowerment is generally defined in reference sources as the granting
of power or authority. Conversely, empowerment can be defined as
the process by which the powerlessness of a stigmatized or oppressed
group (e.g., minorities) is reduced (Lee, 1994). This latter definition
appears to be more applicable to the situation of families of residents
of long-term care institutions. Viewing family members as an oppressed
group may be rather extreme; however, they certainly may experience
feelings of powerlessness when interfacing with the staff at long-term
care institutions. Once the primary duties of caregiving are relinquished
to facility staff, family members may feel that they lack input in decision
making and that they are powerless to effect change in the institution
(Ingersoll-Dayton, Schroepfer, Pryce, & Waarala, 2003). In addition,
family members may be reluctant to express their opinions and concerns because they fear retribution against either themselves or the
residents. Finally, family members who experience inadequate care
may feel powerless to move residents to another facility because they
may be encumbered financially and concerned with the negative
sequelae that often accompany the relocation of an older adult. Prior
to the establishment of family councils, family members had little or
no formal mechanism for freely voicing opinions and concerns. Family
councils fill this need by offering a safe forum for family members
to express their concerns and a process through which concerns are
addressed. By empowering families, family councils help to reduce
some of the powerlessness of having a relative in the institutional setting.

Advocacy

As addressed in the previous section, the advocacy function of family
councils is to address problems and concerns, to interface with the

institution and legislative bodies to effect change, and to provide a voice for residents who are unable to do so for themselves. Family council advocacy operates on three levels: the individual level, the institutional level, and the legislative level (Hepworth, Rooney, & Larsen, 1997). On the individual level, advocates work to secure services and resources for people who are unable to gain access to these means. In the nursing home, family councils advocate on behalf of either individual residents or family members to meet their specific needs and provide these individuals with the knowledge and processes to address their concerns (e.g., expanding programs for a Spanish-speaking resident or family). On the institutional level, family councils work to modify policies and procedures, such as working with the institution to expand formal visiting hours. Family councils also advocate on the legislative level by organizing and lobbying for laws and funding aimed at improving the quality of life for older adults in long-term care.

Support

The support function of family councils is grounded in several concepts drawn from group processes. In addition to the social support that is shared by family council members, individuals may also benefit from the psychotherapeutic aspects of group work (Cox & Ephross, 1989; Yalom, 1975). Over time, family councils develop cohesiveness that bolsters feelings of acceptance and belonging. By sharing problems with the group, family members may feel reassured that they are not alone and that they share many of the same problems and concerns. Family council meetings are also a forum for interpersonal input and output, allowing family members to share information in a nonthreatening environment. Through the exchange of ideas, experiences, and concerns, family councils provide members with a chance for catharsis—an emotional release that allows an individual to achieve balance. Finally, the group meetings may instill hope for family members that they can maintain an active and productive role in the lives of their relatives living in long-term care facilities.

EFFICACY OF FAMILY COUNCILS

Family councils can offer a number of potential benefits for residents and family members, as discussed in the previous section, but institutions and the long-term care industry also benefit from them. As already described, family councils can improve the quality of residents' lives and enhance their well-being as well as provide family members with support, information, and the chance to assume a potentially powerful and positive role in the lives of their relatives. The benefits of family councils for institutions and staff include providing an effective means of communicating concerns and problems and offering a direct pipeline for addressing issues before they must be handled "out of house" (e.g., via the ombudsman, through the legal system). In addition, family councils often offer novel solutions and fresh perspectives that can improve programs, alter policies, and aid the institution in providing quality care. Family councils can also effect change on a policy level by educating and organizing legislators and voters on issues that affect older adults and the care provided in long-term residential facilities (Grant, 2003).

The potential benefits of family councils are numerous and far reaching. However, research on family councils is scant and consists of a handful of articles presenting either anecdotal evidence or the findings from small-scale studies. In short, virtually no empirical evidence either supports or disputes the efficacy of family councils in yielding these positive outcomes. As the previous and subsequent chapters in this book attest, a number of studies have examined family involvement and the roles, perceptions, and interactions of families and staff in long-term care. Yet, a comprehensive database search and review of the literature failed to uncover a quantitative study specifically examining the effects of family councils in their current manifestation. Although the research reviewed here provides a degree of insight into the functioning and impact of family councils, there is considerable need for empirical research to further elucidate the effects of family councils in long-term care.

Palmer (1991) chronicled the conception and effects of a family council in one long-term care facility soon after the OBRA 1987 mandate. The meetings were co-led by a staff social worker and a family member and were well attended by 20–25 family members. Analysis of feedback from family council members 8 months after conception revealed that the meetings were a good source of support and allowed family members to share their experiences in a comfortable environment. Council members indicated that they felt the meetings were helpful and that staff members were cooperative and interested in their concerns. Although these findings point to the potential efficacy of family councils, the cross-sectional design and small scale of this study limit generalizability.

Schwartzben (1992) investigated the evolution and functioning of a family council on one floor of a long-term care institution. (*Note:* Schwartzben used the term *multifamily group,* yet the structure and goals of the group were consistent with that of a family council.) The family council was facilitated by a social worker, and, over an 18-month period, the group grew from 14 to 27 members. Schwartzben identified five general activities of the group: 1) sharing information and mutual support, 2) negotiating the institutional system, 3) sharing information and providing education, 4) communicating and addressing concerns with staff, and 5) planning and supporting social programs and holiday activities. Although no definite methodology was employed to evaluate the family council, the study concluded that the group was successful in helping family members to actively adjust to new roles following admission of their relatives to the institution.

The National Citizens' Coalition for Nursing Home Reform (NCCNHR, 1998) surveyed state and regional ombudsmen and long-term care family advocacy groups in an effort to examine family involvement and, more specifically, the efficacy of family councils. The researchers found that family councils provided a unified voice for families; increased the efficiency of ombudsman work; and gave family members greater respect, credibility, and responsibility in the lives of their relatives. Wide diversity was found in the structure, goals, and overall effectiveness of the family councils. Groups that had strong, consistent leadership and took a positive, constructive approach to problem solving appeared to be more effective. Respondents also reported widespread resistance on the part of facilities. Reported resistance was both passive and active—for example, failing to provide adequate meeting space, promising and then failing to send out meeting reminders to families, and misidentifying family appreciation nights as family council meetings in order to fulfill the legislative requirement to support a family council while avoiding the "hassles" of an actual family council.

The findings from these few studies suggest that the effectiveness of family councils is predicated on a number of factors, including active participation, strong organization, consistent leadership, a constructive approach, and support and cooperation from the facility. Several groups have focused on the characteristics of successful family councils, and actively facilitate and encourage their development in long-term care facilities. In the United States, the NCCNHR has been an ardent supporter of family involvement in long-term care and provides training and resources for families and institutions interested in forming a group.

In Canada, the Family Councils Project has been instrumental in the proliferation of family councils across Ontario. Research that incorporates both qualitative and quantitative elements across a large number of institutions would provide these groups with greater focus and a more stable foundation. In addition, research that compares or combines the work of family councils with other interventions (e.g., staff–family education, cooperation programs) may help to determine the most effective method of achieving the ultimate goal of family councils: improving the lives of residents in long-term care.

A BEST PRACTICE APPROACH TO ORGANIZING AND MAINTAINING A FAMILY COUNCIL

Although family councils are present in many of the long-term care facilities in the United States and Canada, a number of facilities remain without family councils or have family councils that are ineffective or inactive. The following guide to organizing and maintaining a family council in residential long-term care serves as an outline for family members, administrators, and staff. The best practice approach presented here is equally applicable to staff and family members interested in forming a family council. Significant portions of this guide are based on two primary sources: *Family Guide to Effective Family Councils* (Grant, 2003) and *Family Councils in Action* (Hart et al., 1994). Interested readers should refer to these sources for further information and resources that might assist with organizing and maintaining a family council.

Enlisting Support and Providing Information

Despite the efforts of family advocacy groups to disseminate information, many family members are unaware of the presence and functions of family councils in residential long-term care. Therefore, the first step in organizing a family council is to enlist the cooperation of families, residents, and staff and to educate these groups on the nature, functioning, and potential benefits of family councils. Grant (2003) suggested the following steps during the nascent stages of family council development:

- *Connect with family members and residents.* Share the idea and concept of the family council and enlist their support to recruit other family members as potential participants.

- *Contact the long-term care ombudsman in the local Area Agency on Aging.* The ombudsman can serve as a powerful advocate and a good source of information regarding families' rights and the functioning of successful family councils.

- *Connect with family councils in other facilities.* Other family councils can share their experiences and prevent you from having to "re-invent the wheel."

- *Meet with the facility administrator.* Gaining the cooperation of the facility administrator is an important step in organizing a family council. Administrators can facilitate family councils by encouraging cooperation of staff, affording the group adequate meeting space, and ensuring that the concerns of the group are taken seriously. Occasionally, administrators resist the formation of family councils, so it is important to present the rights, goals, and potential benefits to the administrator in an organized, well-prepared, and substantiated manner. If resistance is encountered, then attempt to discuss the concerns with the administrator. If this fails, then the long-term care ombudsman can be contacted to intervene on behalf of the fledgling family council.

Introductory Meeting

After garnering support and providing information, it is essential to hold an introductory meeting to which all families are invited. The purpose of this meeting is to explain the concept of the family council to the larger audience, find out which family members are interested in serving on the council, and begin planning for the first official meeting. It is important to promote the introductory meeting to the widest audience. When possible, families should be contacted via telephone and written invitations. In addition, fliers and posters should be placed around the facility, encouraging all families and residents to attend. The long-term care ombudsman can also be invited and may provide guidance if questions arise. Hart et al. (1994) outlined six tasks to be completed in the introductory meeting:

1. Define and explain the essential characteristics of family councils.

2. Facilitate an atmosphere in which family members can freely discuss their ideas and concerns.

3. Determine if all family members should attend meetings or if a smaller number of family members should serve as representatives. This decision is predicated on the number of people interested in attending.

4. Determine if the family members would like to have a staff member or a resident representative present at the meetings. It is important to note that the attendance of staff and residents at these council meetings can be problematic and may inhibit the free exchange of concerns and ideas between family members. Some family councils avoid problems by appointing staff and resident liaisons who do not attend meetings but who regularly meet with council members to remain informed.

5. Select leaders. This may be done on a temporary basis until the council is better established.

6. Plan for the next meeting by establishing a date, time, place, and topic.

Building the Structure of the Family Council

Following the introductory meeting, the business and structure of the family council can begin to take shape. The agenda for the first official meeting is important because it establishes a number of the fundamental characteristics of the family council. Grant (2003) and Hart et al. (1994) suggested the following agenda for the first meeting:

• Review the functions, rights, and benefits of the family council. The ombudsman, if he or she is in attendance, or the staff liaison may do this.

• Review the proposed leadership structure and the roles and responsibilities of each position. Leadership structure tends to vary across institutions. Staff members, either on a temporary or a permanent basis, lead some family councils. These staff members may play active roles in leading discussions and presenting issues, or they may play a more passive role by simply recording and forwarding the concerns of the council to the nursing home administration. It is suggested that the staff leadership position eventually be phased out as family members become more comfortable in the functioning of the family councils and the leadership roles (Hart et al., 1994; LaBrake, 1996). Others suggest co-leadership between a staff member (usually the facility social worker) and a family member. Co-leadership can augment the problem-solving potential of the group by presenting different perspectives and providing a good example to the group of family–staff cooperation (Palmer, 1991). Effective communication and relationship skills are essential to the success of the co-leadership model, and much depends on the personalities of the leaders and the council members. Finally, family councils can be self-led, with staff serving in a passive capacity, often excluded from meetings. Elections for the leadership and officer positions of the family council should be held after a few meetings have taken place. This will allow leaders to emerge and family members to get to know the personalities and communication styles of each council member.

- Formulate a mission statement and bylaws for the family council. The development of these elements will help the family council operate in a consistent manner and conduct business efficiently and fairly. Once again, the ombudsman can help with this by providing examples of other family councils' mission statements and bylaws (see Hart et al., 1994, pp. 23–26).

- Discuss the approach that the family council will use to communicate and track the progress of issues and concerns. The family council needs to establish the best methods for communicating with the administrator, staff, fellow council members, and residents. It is suggested that concerns directed toward the administrator be in written form to facilitate tracking and to leave a paper trail for follow-up actions. Council members may choose to communicate via a number of means, including suggestion boxes, family council bulletin boards, telephone trees, and e-mail Listservs (Grant, 2003). Communicating with the residents can be accomplished by having a family council representative address the resident council or by inviting a representative of the resident council to selected portions of family council meetings.

- Discuss options for funding the activities of the family council. Although not obligated to assist financially with the operations of the family council, facilities may provide family councils with small budgets for refreshments, supplies, and, in some cases, family appreciation banquets. Other funding sources include donations and fundraisers, such as used book sales and craft and bake sales.

Conducting the Business of the Family Council

Once firmly established, the family council can begin to conduct the functions of the group. One of the central functions of family councils is *providing mutual support*. Family members grapple with a number of emotional challenges (e.g., loss, guilt, anger) when a relative requires the care of a nursing home. These challenges are often further complicated by the challenges imposed by the institution (e.g., relinquishing control, financial burdens). Family councils can provide a venue in which family members can express and share these emotions and find comfort in knowing that they are not alone in their distress. Grant (2003) suggested that a block of time be set aside at the end of each family council meeting to allow family members to express their feelings and concerns.

Although family councils are not intended to take the place of formal support groups, they can help to organize formal support groups that are separate from the family council. As Hart et al. (1994) noted, "Family councils have initiated formal support groups, and formal support groups have led to the formation of family councils. Although councils and support groups are compatible efforts, they are different kinds of organizations" (p. 56). Support groups tend to focus on support only and are generally led by a person trained in facilitating groups (see Chapter 5). In contrast, family councils have multiple foci (e.g., education, advocacy) and are generally led by family members themselves.

An important element of the support function of family councils is connecting with new family members and orienting them to the nursing home. For family members, admission of a relative to a nursing home can be a traumatic and confusing experience. The family council is an ideal vehicle by which to provide information about a number of topics that may not appear evident to family members new to the nursing home environment (e.g., tips for interacting with staff, how laundry services operate). Contacting new family members may be difficult because of confidentiality concerns; however, admissions staff usually will notify new families of the presence and functions of the family council. Family councils may augment these efforts by including information packets with the admissions paperwork, posting signs, and conducting orientation meetings for new family members. Connecting with new family members is essential to the maintenance of an active and effective family council because these individuals take the place of family members who leave the council as a result of the discharge or death of their relatives.

The second function of family councils—*education and dissemination of information*—is closely related to the support and orientation functions described previously. Educating family members can occur through a number of avenues and activities, such as inviting speakers (e.g., the long-term care ombudsman, elder law professionals), presenting videos on disease processes, and distributing printed information. Inviting the facility administrator or a department head (e.g., nursing, housekeeping) to a family council meeting can provide family members with information and insight into the responsibilities and challenges that these professionals face in the long-term care environment. In addition, these meetings can allow family members to establish relationships with the department heads and the administrator, thereby replacing titles with names and faces. Inviting an expert on group processes or organizing a meeting with other family councils in the area are other ideas that can educate council members and help the group to function more effectively (Hart ct al., 1994).

Advocacy and problem solving are two of the most important functions of the family council. "By joining together, families can be a united voice in a united effort . . . it can be easy to ignore one person; it is much harder to ignore a group of people" (Grant, 2003, p. 30). Collective action on issues that concern family members and residents can be a powerful tool for change. However, the approach and method by which the family council expresses concerns play a central role in whether the concern will be acted on and the desired results will be achieved. Although there are several different approaches to problem solving, the following stepwise approach is tailored to family councils and the structure of the nursing home environment (Grant, 2003):

1. Identify a specific problem or concern that is shared by members of the council or that has been reported to be a common problem for other family members in the facility. Collect as much information about the problem as possible, including frequency; past efforts to address the problem; and statements from residents, family members, and staff members.

2. Develop a concise, concrete written problem statement.

3. Identify the objectives that the family council is hoping to achieve.

4. Identify potential solutions to the problem. For example, if the problem deals with lack of variety on the dinner menu, then one solution may be to have an alternative entrée offered each night. It is important to offer creative, realistic solutions rather than simply stating a concern. Without a solution, a problem can take on negative connotations and may be heard by the facility as a complaint rather than a concern.

5. Identify potential barriers that may interfere with achieving the family council's objectives. In the case of the menu example, the facility may reply that it cannot offer an alternative entrée because of costs. The family council should anticipate these arguments and be prepared to offer creative solutions.

6. Develop a plan of action that includes determining who is going to initiate the concern, determining to whom the concern is addressed, and preparing a written statement that incorporates both the concern and the proposed solution(s).

7. Initiate the plan of action. Depending on the nature of the concern, this can vary from simply forwarding the written concern to the staff liaison to meeting with the facility administrator. In the latter case, a family council member should succinctly present the concern, offer possible solutions, and convey the notion that family members are willing to work with the facility in addressing this concern and solving the problem. Whenever possible, a course of action and a time frame for initiating the action should be agreed on at the meeting. Following the meeting, the family council should draft a summary of the meeting with the agreed-on course of action and forward this to the administrator.

8. Monitor the progress of the resolution of the concern. If delays or obstacles become apparent, then schedule another meeting with the administrator to attempt to circumvent these barriers.

9. Evaluate the results of the problem-solving process. If the problem has been successfully resolved, then share this success with other family members, staff, residents, and the administrator. If the problem persists, then continue to work within the family council and

with the administrator to determine alternative approaches. If, over time, the family council encounters persistent difficulty or resistance to solving the problem, then it may be appropriate to contact the long-term care ombudsman for assistance.

Throughout the problem-solving process, it is essential that the family council attempt to establish and foster a positive, symbiotic relationship with the facility staff and administrator. Although this is not possible to achieve in all situations, cooperation and patience are usually the keys to the family council's success in facilitating change. As Grant noted, "Don't expect immediate results. Problems that did not develop overnight usually can't be fixed overnight either" (2003, p. 34).

The advocacy and problem-solving functions of family councils can also be applied to the initiation and processes of legislative action. Certain issues (e.g., mandatory staffing levels) are beyond the scope of advocacy on the institutional level and require family councils to advocate at the state and federal levels. In such cases, family councils can have a positive impact on the quality of life in long-term care settings not only in their own respective facilities but also industrywide. Several steps are suggested to successfully lobby for legislative action (Hart et al., 1994):

- Research and define in writing the problem and the proposed changes. Gathering support and information from residents, family members, other family councils, and advocacy agencies (e.g., AARP, NCCNHR) can be beneficial because it indicates that the problem is pandemic, not facility specific. The services of the long-term care ombudsman may augment these efforts.

- Identify, contact, and attempt to schedule a meeting with the target legislators as early as possible.

- Prepare an organized, concise presentation of the proposed legislative action prior to the meeting. Selected testimony of residents and family members can be very effective in conveying the "human side of the story."

- Follow and support the legislative action as it makes its way through the political process. If possible, attend meetings, conduct telephone and mail campaigns, and aggressively seek media coverage.

- Finally, encourage and facilitate voting among the residents, family members, and staff. Together, this group can be a force for positive change in residential long-term care.

Although family councils often deal with the negative aspects of institutionalization, these groups can also enhance life in the facility through more positive approaches. *Organizing and promoting projects and activities* is a central function of family councils. This function not only enhances the lives of residents, family members, and staff but also builds and strengthens relationships between the facility and the community. Projects that can directly benefit the residents include raising funds to purchase items that improve the environment in the facility (e.g., audiovisual equipment, books, plants), organizing a gift cart that delivers items to residents' rooms, raising funds to provide transportation to activities outside of the facility, and working with the facility and community groups to organize an active volunteer program. Projects directed toward family members include periodic orientation and welcoming receptions for new family members, organizing family support groups, and publishing a newsletter for families. Finally, projects that benefit staff and strengthen the relationships between residents, families, and staff include organizing staff appreciation and recognition events, collaborating on projects with the resident council, and assisting the administration in developing new policies and programs (Grant, 2003; Hart et al., 1994). By assuming a positive role in the nursing home, the family council can ease adversarial tension and encourage cooperation between family members and staff.

Troubleshooting for Family Councils

Although family councils may encounter a range of specific problems, three types of obstacles generally impede the ability of family councils to achieve their goals: lack of participation, dysfunction within the processes of the group, and resistance from the facility (Grant, 2003; Hart et al., 1994). For each type of obstacle, family councils can implement a number of potential solutions. In situations in which problems are persistent, the family council should enlist the expertise of the long-term care ombudsman and contact other family councils to develop effective solutions.

Lack of participation can be a problem for both new and established family councils. Several approaches can be taken to address this problem:

- Redoubling efforts to promote the family council and to recruit participants through orientation packets, posters and fliers, mailing lists, telephone calls, e-mails, receptions, and personal communication with other family members. Creative approaches that have been effective in the past include posting notices on cars outside of the facility a few nights before the next meeting, sponsoring a tea or a cookout, and publicizing meetings in local newspapers and in the local media (e.g., public television and radio) (Grant, 2003).

- Scheduling council meetings at different times of the day to accommodate family members who are employed and family members who are unable to travel in the evening hours

- Revitalizing interest in the family council by selecting goals and projects that are unique, innovative, and, most important, achievable. Success tends to breed success, and family councils that are most effective are the ones that achieve stated goals. Projects that are usually well attended and successful include workshops on estate planning; presentations on Medicare, Medicaid, and insurance issues; and events that are covered by the local media (NCCNHR, 1998).

Problems related to group processes include ineffective meetings, lack of leadership, and lack of understanding of effective collective action. Potential solutions include

- Ensuring that the group adheres to the set agenda at meetings. This will enable the group to remain organized and effectively process identified concerns.

- Routing individuals who dominate meetings with their own concerns through the proper channels in order to expedite the problem-solving process. Note, however, that the individual problem may actually be a problem that other family members are experiencing. If so, then the group should place this item on the agenda and handle it according to council policy.

- Ensuring that the council members and leaders understand their roles and responsibilities. The ombudsman can provide an in-service on this topic and help to reestablish working order to a wayward family council.

- Inviting an expert on advocacy and group processes to a meeting to provide training to the council members on the mechanisms of collective action

On occasion, family councils may experience resistance from the facility in organizing and problem solving. In such cases, the family council has a number of options:

- Meeting with the administrator to explain and reassert the purposes, goals, and rights of the family council. Maintain a positive, cooperative approach, and attempt to "sell" the benefits of the family council to the facility.

- Contacting the long-term care ombudsman to report the difficulties that the family council has experienced. It is important to have the episodes of facility resistance well documented when presenting the case to the ombudsman. The ombudsman can then recommend a course of action that is appropriate for the situation.

- Seeking legal action. This should be a last resort for family councils when facility resistance is encountered. Maintaining a working relationship with the facility is essential, and legal action against the facility can contaminate this association and hinder future efforts to work in collaboration with the facility. Nevertheless, legal action remains an option that is appropriate in extreme situations.

CONCLUSION

Families who relinquish primary care responsibilities to long-term care institutions enter into a system that can be confusing, frustrating, and less than ideal in terms of the services provided to both residents and families. Family councils can provide orientation and support for family members as they endure this time of change and also serve as a powerful vehicle to enhance communication and advocacy for residents, family members, and nursing home staff. As residential long-term care becomes a reality for more and more individuals and families, family councils may emerge as significant sources of support, advocacy, and empowerment. With this increased focus, there will be an accompanying need for additional research on the elements that add to and detract from the success of family councils in residential long-term care. Through additional research and advocacy efforts, family councils should continue to be an outlet, resource, and catalyst for family involvement and change in long-term care.

REFERENCES

Aneshensel, C.S., Pearlin, L.I., Mullan, J.T., Zarit, S.H., & Whitlatch, C.J. (1995). *Profiles in caregiving: The unexpected career.* San Diego: Academic Press.

Bailey, P., & Poole, J. (2004). *Families in long-term care: A brief review of the literature.* Retrieved February 17, 2004, from http://www.familycouncils.net/lit.html

Cox, C., & Ephross, P.H. (1989). Group work with families of nursing home residents: Its socialization and therapeutic functions. *Journal of Gerontological Social Work, 13*(3/4), 61–73.

Grant, R. (2003). *Family guide to effective family councils.* Chicago: Legal Assistance Foundation of Metropolitan Chicago.

Hart, M., Rehwaldt, M., & Clark, E. (1994). *Family councils in action: A manual for organizing and developing family councils in nursing and boarding care homes.* Minneapolis: Minnesota Alliance for Health Care Consumers.

Hepworth, D.H., Rooney, R.H., & Larsen, J.A. (1997). *Direct social work practice: Theory and skills* (5th ed.). Pacific Grove, CA: Brooks/Cole.

Hertzberg, A., & Ekman, S.L. (1996). How the relatives of elderly patients in institutional care perceive the staff. *Scandinavian Journal of Caring Sciences, 10,* 205–211.

Hook, W.F., Sobal, J., & Oak, J.C. (1982). Frequency of visitation in nursing homes: Patterns of contact across barriers in total institutions. *The Gerontologist, 22,* 424–428.

Ingersoll-Dayton, B., Schroepfer, T., Pryce, J., & Waarala, C. (2003). Enhancing relationships in nursing homes through empowerment. *Social Work, 48,* 420–424.

LaBrake, T. (1996). *How to get families more involved in the nursing home: Four programs that work and why.* New York: Haworth.

Lee, J.A.B. (1994). *The empowerment approach to social work practice.* New York: Columbia University Press.

National Citizens' Coalition for Nursing Home Reform. (1998). *Family education and outreach: Final report.* Washington, DC: Author.

Omnibus Budget Reconciliation Act (OBRA) of 1987, PL 100-203, 42 U.S.C.

Palmer, D.S. (1991). Co-leading a family council in a long-term care facility. *Journal of Gerontological Social Work, 16*(3/4), 121–134.

Pillemer, K. (1996). *Solving the frontline crisis in long-term care.* Albany, NY: Delmar/Thompson.

Ross, M.M., Rosenthal, C.J., & Dawson, P. (1997). Spousal caregiving in the institutional setting: Visiting. *Journal of Clinical Nursing, 6,* 473–483.

Rowles, G.D., & High, D.M. (1996). Individualized care: Family roles in nursing home decision-making. *Journal of Gerontological Nursing, 22*(3), 20–25.

Schwartzben, S.H. (1992). Social work with multi-family groups: A partnership model for long term care settings. *Social Work in Health Care, 18*(1), 23–38.

Smith, K., & Bengtson, V. (1979). Positive consequences of institutionalization: Solidarity between elderly parents and their middle-aged children. *The Gerontologist, 19,* 438–447.

Tornatore, J.B., & Grant, L.A. (2004). Family caregiver satisfaction with the
    nursing home after placement of a relative with dementia. *Journals of Geron-
    tology. Series B, Psychological Sciences and Social Sciences, 59,* S80–S88.
Yalom, I.D. (1975). *The theory and practice of group psychotherapy.* New York:
    Basic Books.
York, J.L., & Calsyn, R.J. (1977). Family involvement in nursing homes. *The
    Gerontologist, 17,* 500–505.

RESOURCES

For additional assistance in identifying resources to assist in the development or operation of a family council, please contact

> Keith A. Anderson, M.S.W.
> Graduate Center for Gerontology
> The University of Kentucky
> 306 Health Sciences Building
> 900 S. Limestone
> Lexington, KY 40536
> E-mail: kaande3@uky.edu
> Telephone: 859-257-1450, ext. 80184

In addition to the text and references included in this chapter, the
following resources may be of assistance to healthcare professionals,
family members, and residents of long-term care who are interested
in establishing or strengthening family councils in their facilities:

National Citizens' Coalition for Nursing Home Reform (NCCNHR)
1828 L Street, NW
Suite 801
Washington, DC 20036
Telephone: 202-332-2275
http://www.nccnhr.org

National Long-Term Care Ombudsman Resource Center
1828 L Street, NW
Suite 801
Washington, DC 20036
Telephone: 202-332-2275
http://www.ltcombudsman.org

Ontario Family Councils Program
40 Orchard View Boulevard
Suite 219
Toronto, ON M4R1B9
Telephone: 888-283-8806
http://www.familycouncils.net

3

Promoting Family Involvement in Long-Term Care

A Certified Nursing Assistant's Perspective

KATHERINA A. NIKZAD

Family involvement is such an individual matter. There are so many factors involved severity of illness, length of illness, age, health and ability of caregivers, proximity to facility. I have observed so many different situations. Some people cannot tolerate seeing their loved ones in confinement; therefore, they visit rarely, if at all. Some people are no longer physically able to actively participate in the resident's care. Some, unfortunately, are in denial and do not want to face the situation of their loved one having Alzheimer's disease.

I should think that there would be a fine line to tread when attempting to further family involvement. People may welcome suggestions but may feel they have transferred caregiving responsibilities to the facilities, therefore relinquishing caregiving entirely. The question is, how do you get families to stay involved after their loved one is no longer living with them?

—Wife of a man with Alzheimer's disease
living in a long-term care facility

Admission to a long-term care facility may occur for a variety of reasons, most commonly because of age-related illnesses or complications that create barriers for individuals to remain living independently in their homes. Admitting a family member to a long-term care facility creates many transitions for family caregivers, who often serve as the main informal (unpaid) care providers for older individuals with disabilities (Gaugler, Leitsch, Zarit, & Pearlin, 2000; Hansson et al., 1990). Once admission occurs, family members no longer find themselves in the role of the primary caregiver. This role transition, however, does not mark the end of family involvement in the lives of elderly relatives. Research over the years has demonstrated that family involvement in the lives and care procedures of elderly relatives does not cease following the admission of an older individual to residential care (e.g., Davis & Buckwalter, 2001; Gaugler et al., 2000; Naleppa, 1996). In contrast, family members, although no longer considered primary caregivers, often continue their involvement in the lives of elderly relatives who reside in long-term care settings. Furthermore, research has shown that family members continue to feel a need to be involved in the lives of older relatives and to sustain their role as a care provider, however minimal (Tickle & Hull, 1995).

Barriers exist for some family members when it comes to maintaining a level of postadmission involvement, however. Prior to admitting their relative to a long-term care facility, family caregivers, especially those caring for individuals with Alzheimer's disease (AD), are highly prone to adverse mental and physical health complications, such as stress, fatigue, burnout, depression, and loneliness (Annerstedt, Elmstahl, Ingvad, & Samuelsson, 2000; Pinquart & Sorensen, 2003a, 2003b; Silliman & Sternberg, 1988; Vitaliano, Zhang, & Scanlan, 2003). In a study conducted by Gaugler et al. (2000), the researchers found that older individuals who exhibited negative and problematic behaviors prior to their admission to long-term care received fewer postadmission visits from family members, who may have wished to avoid additional stress caused by these severe behavior problems. For reasons such as these, it becomes extremely important to develop strategies to effectively involve family members in the lives of their elderly relatives following institutionalization.

Because admitting a family member to a nursing facility brings about many changes for both family members and residents, it is important to recognize and utilize ways to promote continued family involvement following admission. This process can be enhanced through the combined efforts of formal caregivers (i.e., nursing home staff) and informal caregivers (i.e., family members, close friends), who each play a role in the level of involvement in the lives of nursing home residents. Strategies for promoting family involvement in long-term care may be more effective when family members and formal caregivers work together to enhance the type of involvement that will provide the most successful outcomes for both the elderly resident and his or her family members. Certified nursing assistants (CNAs) typically spend the greatest amount of time with residents and provide the majority of personal care (e.g., bathing, feeding, dressing, transferring). Now placed in the role of primary caregivers, CNAs have the capacity to encourage and promote a continuation of family involvement during and after the admission process in a variety of ways.

The goal of this chapter is to provide insight regarding the importance of family involvement and to offer ways to enhance involvement through a variety of effective strategies that could be utilized and evaluated in long-term care settings. These strategies include effective interaction between nursing home staff and family members, conveying important information to family members regarding resident status, informing family members of upcoming activities to participate in, and teaching family members effective communication strategies to use when interacting with patients with AD and other types of dementia. Each of these strategies is derived from a CNA perspective and is supplemented with in-depth accounts from family members who reveal their personal experiences of placing a relative in a nursing home.

INTERACTING WITH FAMILY MEMBERS

As staff members in a long-term care facility, CNAs inevitably interact with family members. Because they have the greatest amount of contact with older residents, CNAs are involved in many situations in which they need to communicate directly with family members regarding a variety of topics and concerns. For example, if a resident becomes ill or is demonstrating signs of depression, withdrawal, changes in appetite, or mood alterations, CNAs are typically the first ones to identify such changes and are responsible for making families aware of these episodes. Likewise, if incidents between two residents continually occur (e.g., arguments, inappropriate behavior), families should be informed so they can intervene if needed. Therefore, the first strategy that should be utilized by staff to promote a family member's involvement is the process of actively associating with visiting family members and doing so in a way that is deemed appropriate and effective.

There are several approaches that a CNA can take in order to associate successfully with family members. Upon an older individual's admission to a long-term care facility, families may remain hesitant or unaware of what to expect from the facility or staff during the first few months. Establishing a sense of rapport and security with those closest to the resident must be accomplished first in order to progress through the next stages of successful communication. For example, CNAs can acknowledge family members when they arrive for visits and make the effort of introducing themselves as caregivers. Acknowledging the presence of family members and taking the time to initiate conversations offers a sense of belonging and trust between families and primary care staff members. In addition, staff interactions and behaviors will have a great impact on the family's perceptions of the nursing home environment (Riddick, Cohen-Mansfield, Fleshner, & Kraft, 1992). Once a family member begins to feel comfortable and welcome in the nursing home setting, he or she may feel more inclined to continue his or her visits.

Once trust is established between families and staff, CNAs should strongly advise families to continue to make decisions for their relatives by asking for the input and opinions of family members. This can be accomplished by allowing families to have equal speaking time during conversations and through dual decision making. This process of interacting with family members allows both the staff and the family to directly express their concerns and requests regarding residents (e.g., clothing, food preferences, behavioral concerns). This type of communication is reciprocal in nature in that both the families and staff are contributing equally to the care that will be provided for the resident. Agreement among staff and family members, as demonstrated in the sample CNA–family interaction that follows, not only helps to create a more stable and effective environment for the residents but also encourages a continuation of active involvement from the families, who will attain a more positive outlook on the nursing facility through positive staff interactions.

Adult Son: I am worried that my dad is losing too much weight. He has lost almost 8 pounds within the last month.

CNA: We've noticed that your dad has been more distracted during mealtimes. He does a lot of pacing and fidgeting, and he will only take a few bites before pushing his food away. The other staff and I think this might be happening because your dad doesn't like the food that is on his tray. Do you have any suggestions about the types of food your dad likes to eat?

Adult Son: Dad always loved corn on the cob and roast beef when we were growing up. He prefers a lot of red meat over chicken, and he loves potatoes on the side. He also doesn't like any type of green vegetables. He's been that way since I can remember.

CNA: We are also having trouble getting your dad to drink liquids. Maybe if we offered him different things he would be more willing to drink them. What are some of his favorite things to drink?

Adult Son: He loves orange juice, and he will drink almost every type of soda. He has never liked to drink milk, but if there is chocolate syrup in it he will most likely drink it. Also, he always drank his water with ice cubes in it. He would rarely drink a glass of water if it didn't have ice in it.

CNA: Do you have any other suggestions that might help us get your dad to eat?

Adult Son: Dad was used to a quiet atmosphere when he ate. Maybe if you sat him at a table that was away from the other residents he might be more willing to sit down longer and eat.

CNA: I really appreciate all of your suggestions. I will notify the kitchen this afternoon and request meal changes that might better accommodate your dad's food preferences. The rest of the staff and I will let your dad eat at a quieter setting for dinner tonight. We will let you know if this helps him to start eating more and if he starts to gain some of his weight back.

In this example, the CNA has requested information from the son regarding a problem and has utilized the son's input concerning his father. The CNA has also reassured the son that she will immediately begin new interventions to help his father eat during meals and that the family will be notified if any changes occur. Because a mutual exchange of information and concerns occurred during this conversation, the son is going to feel that his opinion is respected and valued and will feel assured that the problem will be dealt with adequately. This experience will ultimately encourage further involvement from the son.

Once communication consists of trust and mutual exchange of information, CNAs must then be prepared to converse with families during a variety of difficult situations, such as a resident's illness or death. Although social workers and grief counselors typically assume responsibility for families during these circumstances, CNAs are almost always present during the resident's illness and death and need to acquire an understanding of how to interact with families when such a crisis is occurring. In these circumstances, it is crucial for CNAs to be able not only to respond appropriately to a resident's needs but also to offer support and comfort to families who are witnessing a loved one's progressing illness or death process, as expressed by an adult daughter regarding her experience with her mother's death from AD:

> I remember when my mother was dying in the nursing home. It was so awful to watch because all I could do was think, "That's not my mother, that's not the way she used to be." I would sit beside her bed at all hours of night, just waiting for something to happen. The aides on all shifts would continually check in on me and make sure my mother, as well as myself, had everything that we needed. Sometimes it was as simple as one of them bringing me a cup of coffee or just listening to me when I wanted to talk about my mother when she was young and healthy. When Mom finally did pass away, the aides comforted me by hugging me, crying with me, and offering sympathy and prayers. They made sure that Mother looked presentable when the funeral home came for her. I really didn't expect them to do so much, but it was a great comfort to know that these were the people who cared for my mother in her final days.

Interacting with families during difficult situations in long-term care settings is a challenging task, but one that can be accomplished through the efforts of knowledgeable staff workers who are educated and prepared to interact efficiently on a daily basis. Enhancing a family's involvement will be more likely to occur if the communication and interaction taking place is done with mutual respect, a reciprocal exchange of thoughts and concerns, and a level of trust that is evident between staff and family members.

CONVEYING INFORMATION TO FAMILY MEMBERS

Communication with family members also requires the ability to discern what types of information are proper and necessary to convey. Understanding information that should and should not be provided to families is essential and needs to be thoroughly understood by staff in long-term care. Because CNAs spend the majority of their time caring for nursing home residents, they obtain a great deal of information regarding the progress, changes in health, changes in behavior, and changes in cognition of each resident being cared for. Conveying this type of information to family members helps keep them informed of the current health and mental status of their elderly relatives. Moreover, making families aware of the current status of their older relatives may help create a greater sense of familiarity and predictability for families during their personalized visits. An adult daughter whose mother resided in a nursing home until her death from AD noted this need for information:

> If I had it to do all over again, I wish I could have obtained more information from staff members concerning my mother. That way when I went for visits I would have known what to expect from her. The only time the nursing home ever contacted me was when my mother was out of medication. I realize how busy they are during the day, but it would have been wonderful to hear even the smallest things that she did. The disease itself is so negative, and all we ever hear about are the negative things that happen. Every little bit of positive news helps. It would have made my day if I was told that "Hey, your mom smiled today."

Although reporting information to family members is an imperative responsibility of a CNA, an important factor that one also must consider is the type of information that is most relevant to convey and the manner in which to present this information. Some residents, primarily those with AD or other forms of dementia, for example, tend to exhibit behavior problems and verbal disturbances at unpredictable times. Although it is reasonable to make family members aware of this type of behavior, to focus continually on the negative aspects of the resident's behavior may become disturbing and upsetting for some family members. Rather than only make known to families the negative behaviors or occurrences, nursing home staff should place a greater emphasis on the positive attributes exhibited by residents and convey this type of information to family members more often. Highlighting resident achievements, such as self-feeding or improved mobility, is reassuring for family members because it offers them a sense of comfort knowing that their relative is continuing to make progress in different aspects of his or her life.

The following scenario depicts how staff members can communicate information to family members in a more positive manner.

Mrs. Weiland is a resident in a nursing home and is in the middle stages of AD. Her moods and behaviors change periodically, and on this particular day she is upset, irritable, and exhibiting several behavior problems toward staff and other residents. She refused her bath in the morning and reportedly slapped one of the aides across the face when the aide attempted to bathe her. During breakfast, she began screaming and throwing her food, upsetting other residents sitting at the same table. By that afternoon, Mrs. Weiland had calmed down and began quietly pacing the hallways. She cooperated with staff when it was time to sit down for lunch and allowed the aides to shampoo and style her hair following lunch, while engaging in conversation with them. When Mrs. Weiland's adult daughter came in to visit later that day, she saw her mother looking especially nice, and her mother's mood was calm and pleasant. The daughter had repeatedly seen her mother get upset and act violently toward the staff and even toward her. It is difficult for Mrs. Weiland's daughter to see and hear about her mother's negative behavior because these incidents would have never occurred when Mrs. Weiland was healthy. Consider how the aides responded to the daughter's questions about her mother's behavior in the following dialogue.

Daughter: How has mom been acting today?

    CNA: She was a little agitated this morning, so we decided to wait until later in the afternoon to let her have her bath. After breakfast she began feeling a little bit better and she seemed more comfortable around us.

Daughter: Has she been violent at all today?

    CNA: She was a little resistive this morning, but as the day went on she began to relax and we had a nice time together after lunch. She was very talkative while we were fixing her hair, and her speech was especially coherent today.

Daughter: I am so glad that I came today when she is behaving so well. I look forward to days like these when I can come in and spend time with her and not be upset because of the changes in her personality.

In this scenario, the CNA chose to report information to a family member in a way that contains fewer negative implications about the resident's behavior, which could have been frustrating and upsetting for the daughter to hear. Although some negative incidents did occur that day, the staff chose to elaborate on the positive aspects of Mrs. Weiland's behavior (e.g., cooperation with staff, coherent speech). Conveying information in this way is much more tolerable for family members, who have to continually cope with the difficult changes in their relative's moods and behaviors as a result of AD. Focusing on the positive behaviors exhibited by residents with AD and viewing the situation in a more optimistic manner is comforting for families and may encourage their level of involvement in the resident's life.

It is crucial for staff members, especially those having the most contact with residents, to understand the importance of communicating with families and how this communication will ultimately influence family members. Families tend to rely heavily on statements and judgments made by staff, and they place a great deal of trust in what is said about their older relatives. For this reason, staff members have an obligation to ensure that family members receive sufficient information concerning their relatives and that it is done in a way that also protects the emotional well-being of the family.

INFORMING FAMILIES OF UPCOMING ACTIVITIES

Although interaction and communication between staff and family members is a vital component for promoting family involvement, additional steps need to be taken to ensure that families continue to play a role in the lives of their elderly relatives. A simple way of promoting a family member's involvement is to include him or her in ongoing activities provided by the facility (see Table 3.1).

A majority of long-term care facilities provide a variety of activities and entertainment for resident participation on a daily basis. Because family members may no longer have the opportunity to participate in activities with their older relatives outside of the facility, it is important to include families in the activities that occur within the facility. This can be accomplished in several ways. For example, staff can make the effort to invite family members to participate in upcoming events such as musical programs or community outings. Providing family members with monthly calendars containing scheduled daily activities can serve as reminders of upcoming events. When family members are unavailable during daily scheduled activities, making them aware of evening

Table 3.1.   Examples of activities that may encourage family involvement

Activity	Description
Resident-of-the-month luncheon	Each month a resident is chosen as resident of the month. Family members of that resident are invited to the facility to have lunch with their older relative and staff members.
Reminiscing and life review activities	Through the use of stories, photographs, and other memorabilia, these activities (done individually or in group settings) can be therapeutic for both residents and their family members because they offer the opportunity to remember past events and to engage in meaningful conversation.
Family picnics	Picnics hosted by the facility allow families to enjoy outdoor socialization with their relatives and to interact with other visiting families.
Holiday celebrations	Families are invited to participate in holiday celebrations (e.g., Christmas, Thanksgiving, Valentine's Day) hosted by the facility. These activities are especially valuable for spouses to spend quality time together as a couple.
Musical activities	Musical entertainment offers families the opportunity to come to the facility and enjoy various musical programs performed by members in the community (e.g., church choirs, barbershop quartets). Musical activities are highly encouraged for individuals with Alzheimer's disease because they are soothing and nondemanding.
Spiritual activities	Families are welcome to attend religious services at the facilities and may participate in or help provide music for services. Additional activities include Bible studies, group Rosary, reading the Koran, synagogue services, and other denomination-specific activities.
Group trivia	These cognitively stimulating activities are suitable for participation by both residents and families. Subjects typically include movies, music, literature, and pop culture.

and weekend activities may give them more opportunities to participate. In addition, simply encouraging family members to attend mealtimes in the facility is one way of ensuring that families have the opportunity to stay involved in the lives of long-term care residents.

The manner in which activities are designed will also have an impact on the level of family participation. In order to make activities appealing for families, they must be designed in such a way that families feel welcome and comfortable in the long-term care setting, as one CNA explains:

Activities need to be designed in a way that promotes not only resident participation but also group participation from their families as well. I believe this would make the atmosphere more comfortable for visiting family members. Often, with Alzheimer's disease, it is difficult for visiting family members to participate in one-to-one activities with their older relative, especially when speech loss has occurred. Group activities may offer a greater sense of belonging, as well as the opportunity for different families to bond with one another. It is important for CNAs to encourage group settings and to offer their input on the activities that are being offered.

The more that family members feel welcome to participate in activities with their older relative, the more likely they are to stay involved over time. These simple efforts from staff can help ensure that family members remain active and involved in events that they may otherwise never have the opportunity to partake in.

TEACHING FAMILIES TO COMMUNICATE WITH PATIENTS WITH ALZHEIMER'S DISEASE

Perhaps one of the most crucial aspects of promoting family involvement from a CNA perspective is educating family members about effective forms of communication to use when interacting with elderly relatives during their visits. This issue becomes increasingly relevant when dealing with residents who have various forms of neurodegenerative illnesses, primarily AD, which cause numerous cognitive and physical losses, bringing about myriad challenges for both the resident with AD and his or her family members (Cohen, 1999).

One of the main barriers affecting residents with AD and their family members involves communication (Touzinsky, 1998). Family members of residents with AD report that a majority of their stress is a result of unsuccessful communication between the resident and themselves. This in turn can cause additional psychological stress on the families and the resident (Small, Kemper, & Lyons, 1997). Residents with AD who are unable to successfully communicate their feelings, wants, needs, and fears often experience additional emotional and psychological stress and frustration as a result of this inability (Feil, 1984). Several researchers (e.g., Dippel & Hutton, 1988; Helfer, 1991; Ostuni & Santo-Pietro, 1991) have proposed that improving verbal and nonverbal communication may lead to a reduction in many of the complications that arise, for both the resident and the family members, as a consequence of the disease.

For several decades, reality orientation has served as the primary technique for communicating with individuals with AD. Reality orientation, simply stated, is reorienting a confused individual with dementia to the reality that exists for the caregiver. It is the process of continuously reinforcing orientation to time, place, and person (i.e., present date, year, surroundings, and other individuals). A disadvantage of this approach, however, is that it can potentially cause more harm than benefit when communicating with persons with AD. Because of its structured substance, reality orientation tends to overlook the emotional needs of the individual with AD (O'Donovan, 1996).

People with AD gradually lose their ability to stay oriented to time, place, and person, and many individuals will regress to an earlier time period in their lives (O'Donovan, 1996). It is not uncommon for individuals with AD to speak of a deceased spouse as if he or she were still living. Many will also refer to their children as if they, too, were still infants requiring care. Contradicting these notions with present-day, reality-based information, which many family members are naturally inclined to do, may cause severe damage to their relative's emotional well-being and self-esteem. Smythe and Haworth (1995) reported that implementation of reality orientation in caregiving procedures may even lead to hostility and withdrawal by the person with AD. Because effective communication is extremely important for the well-being of an individual with AD, a need exists for an approach deemed successful and appropriate for family members to use when communicating with their relative with AD.

Awareness of alternative approaches to communicating with individuals with AD is continuing to expand. Validation therapy (VT) is one of these approaches. VT originated in 1963 through the efforts of Naomi Feil, a gerontological social worker, who recognized a need for the development of a method of communication that moved beyond the boundaries of orienting persons with AD to the "here and now" (Day, 1997). VT is based on the belief that the reality experienced by a person diagnosed with AD is as valid and important as if it were our own reality. It assumes the humanistic principle of accepting an individual for his or her uniqueness, even while in the advanced stages of the disease (Woodrow, 1998).

An extremely important principle regarding VT is that an individual with AD should not be judged solely on the behaviors and emotions he or she is displaying throughout the disease process. Rather, each of these behaviors and emotions must be viewed and understood within the context of the person's physical, psychological, and social needs. Thus, VT embraces 10 primary principles (see Table 3.2) that are used to help caregivers better understand what individuals with AD are feeling and why certain behaviors are continually exhibited (Feil, 1992b).

The argument that VT presents is that the actual time of day or year in our own reality is irrelevant when caring for individuals

Table 3.2. Feil's 10 principles of Validation therapy

1. All people are unique and should be treated as individuals.

2. All people are valuable, no matter how disoriented they are.

3. There is a reason behind the behavior of disoriented people.

4. Behavior in old age is not only a function of changes in the brain's anatomy but reflects physical, social, and psychological changes that take place during the lifespan.

5. Behaviors of older people can be changed only if the person wants to change them.

6. Older individuals should be accepted nonjudgmentally.

7. Each stage of life has particular life tasks to be completed. Failure to complete these tasks may lead to psychological problems.

8. When recent memory fails, older adults restore balance to their lives by retrieving memories from the past.

9. Painful feelings that are expressed, acknowledged, and validated by a trusted listener will diminish. Painful feelings that are ignored will gain strength.

10. Empathy builds trust, reduces anxiety, and restores dignity.

From Feil, N. (2003). *The validation breakthrough* (2nd ed., pp. 28–29). Baltimore, MD: Health Professions Press; adapted by permission.

diagnosed with AD. Rather, we should strive to understand and make sense of the reality that the person is experiencing (O'Donovan, 1996). What is important when communicating with individuals with AD is that they feel secure and content within their environment and that those caring for them respect and restore their dignity.

There are several ways to ensure that family members and caregivers use VT techniques properly when they are communicating with individuals with AD. Families should express their emotions in ways that match the emotions of their relative with AD. By doing this, family members are connecting with the feelings experienced by their relative. Rephrasing statements provided by the person with AD in ways that make sense to both the person and his or her family is also a proper validating technique.

Additional techniques include reminiscing and triggering visual memories by looking at family photographs or pictures from magazines. These are several validating procedures that lead to an establishment of rapport and trust between the person with AD and his or her family members. Other techniques used during VT include nonverbal validation techniques such as eye contact, repetitive motions, touch, music, and mirroring when interacting with a person with AD (Day, 1997; Feil, 1993).

Although VT is capable of improving quality of life for both the individual with AD and his or her family members when used appropriately, one must also be cautious in deciding when and with whom VT techniques should be used. Feil (1992a) claimed that VT provides advantages for individuals with AD and some other forms of dementia.

However, those with dementia resulting from psychosis may not respond well to VT techniques. Furthermore, those who are in the early stages of AD, according to Feil (1993), may not benefit from VT because they still possess higher cognitive abilities. Therefore, it becomes crucial that family members have a firm understanding of an individual's diagnosis and are properly educated regarding the uses and advantages of VT.

Two case examples serve to illustrate the appropriate use of VT with residents with AD by staff and family members. In the first, a caregiver uses VT with a resident with AD wanting to leave the nursing home.

Ingrid: Goodbye, everyone. I have to go.

Caregiver: Where are you headed?

Ingrid: Home, of course.

Caregiver: Who do you miss the most at home? (Relating to feelings, using polarity)

Ingrid: My mother, of course.

Caregiver: You feel safe with her?

Ingrid: Of course. She loves me. That's why I have to leave now.

Caregiver: You feel alone here?

Ingrid: I need to go home.

Caregiver: (With empathy) It's hard to be alone, without someone you love?

Ingrid: Yes. (Whispering)

Caregiver: (Gently touching Ingrid's shoulder) Do you miss Edward, too?

Ingrid: Edward loves me. (Her eyes light.)

Caregiver: (Mirroring Ingrid's movements while moving together away from the door) What do you love the most about him? (Reminiscing) His eyes? (Using visual memory)

Ingrid: They are so blue, like my son's.

Caregiver: How did you meet him?

Ingrid has forgotten that she wanted to go home. She feels less lonely. She trusts the caregiver. She cannot go by clock time, but by her memories. Caregiver and Ingrid sing "Let Me Call You Sweetheart" and return to the craft room until Ingrid's husband arrives to take her home.

The second case study is adapted from *The Validation Breakthrough* (Feil, 1993):

Jane's 92-year-old mother was diagnosed as having Alzheimer's disease. She hides her picture albums, her scrapbooks, and her wedding ring, and then she accuses Jane of throwing her precious things away. When Jane finds the ring and the pictures, her mother turns her back on Jane and walks away, muttering, "How did you know where they were? You got them out of the garbage can where you threw them." How should Jane handle this situation?

Answer: Jane should help her mother express her rage and empathize with her fear of aging, dependence, loneliness, and death. Jane needs to understand that her mother's possessions are symbols of her youth. Jane can use the following VT techniques:

Rephrase (builds trust): "Your wedding ring is gone, and you say I have stolen it?"

Use the Visual Sense: "That was that beautiful white gold wedding ring with the date of your marriage engraved on the inside."

Reminisce: "How old were you when you married, Mom? How old was Dad? How did you meet him?"

If Jane genuinely listens to and empathizes with her mother, her mother will tell her how much she has lost. If Jane uses these techniques every day for about 10 minutes, after about 3 weeks her mother's grief will lessen. She will stop hiding her possessions, and she will feel less fearful with Jane because she trusts Jane, who has chosen to listen to and understand her.

Each of these examples demonstrates how families and caregivers can use validating principles in order to handle difficult situations involving an individual with AD. If a family member is unaware of how to handle these situations, he or she will be more likely to withdraw from the relative, and involvement will slowly decline. Educating families with techniques such as VT not only helps them to manage complex situations but allows them to partake in more meaningful conversations and activities with their relatives.

In addition to residents with AD and their family members benefiting from VT, formal caregivers receive many benefits as well. VT has been found to be effective for staff caring for persons with AD living in long-term care settings. Formal caregivers, especially CNAs, are highly prone to great amounts of stress, burnout, and fatigue as a result of rigorous care demands. VT has the capacity to offer staff members relief from these negative consequences by reducing frustration, lowering burnout rates, improving communication, and increasing job satisfaction (Feil, 1993). For example, the Alzheimer's Association (2000) reported a decrease in employee turnover rates and an overall reduction in employee burnout when VT was used during caregiving procedures. When formal caregivers are properly educated and trained to use validating techniques, they are then able to educate family members to do the same in order to help them have more successful and enjoyable visits with their older relatives.

Like any intervention that claims to have a positive impact on psychological functioning, VT has been investigated by several researchers, in both an empirical and an anecdotal manner. A credible strength of the research conducted on VT involves the application of VT sessions in clinical settings and, in most cases, the use of a trained Validation therapist (Bleathman & Morton, 1992).

One attempt to examine the effectiveness of VT was completed by Toseland et al. (1997). These researchers incorporated group VT within a nursing home context and examined its effectiveness in controlling behavior problems and enhancing psychosocial well-being in persons with AD and other types of dementia. Participants were randomly assigned to one of three groups: the Validation therapy group (VT), the social contact group (SC), or the usual care group (UC). Assessments were conducted at baseline, 3 months, and 1 year after group interventions. Results indicated a reduction in verbal and physical aggression in the VT group. However, there was no decrease in nonaggressive problem behaviors in the VT group. An increase in depressive symptoms was found in the SC group, but no changes in depressive symptoms were evident among the UC group. Additionally, those in the SC group experienced a reduction in verbally aggressive behavior. A significant strength in the study was the presence of the SC group. By having the SC group, the researchers were able to rule out the possibility that any changes observed in the VT group were a result of the attention that these residents received during their group sessions.

Because VT claims to have a positive impact on family members, it has been investigated in a more exploratory manner in order to demonstrate its effectiveness for the family. In work conducted by Touzinsky (1998), VT was explored through the use of a case study. The interaction between a man with middle-stage AD and his daughter was observed for several months. The daughter was taught how to use validating techniques rather than her usual reorienting strategies. Within weeks of using VT, the daughter reported significant changes in her father's mood, as well as a decrease in her own depressive symptoms that had resulted from her father's agitation. Through her utilization of VT, the relationship between the father and daughter improved, as did the emotional welfare of both.

For decades, family members and staff have continued to support the efficacy of VT through personal accounts of experiencing fewer communication barriers and reduced caregiver burden, and witnessing an improvement in resident well-being. Family visits have the potential to become more enjoyable and meaningful when proper communication techniques are utilized. When a family member is educated regarding the most effective ways to communicate with his or her relative with AD, he or she is less likely to experience many of the negative outcomes associated with having a relative with this disease. Because of their many benefits for family members, residents, and staff, VT and other effectual communication techniques in the care of individuals with AD are approaches that CNAs are strongly encouraged to employ in order to help promote family involvement.

IMPLEMENTATION AND EVALUATION OF STRATEGIES

Although ways to promote family involvement can be debated and discussed, it is the actual process of implementing these strategies and evaluating their effectiveness that remains truly the most important component to promoting family involvement. If promoting family involvement is to be accomplished successfully, then the best way of obtaining ideas for strategies is to consider the needs of the family members and utilize their input. Suggestions for promoting family involvement presented by family members of residents with AD living in long-term care facilities include the following:

1. Let it be known that involvement of family and friends is important, welcomed, and appreciated.

2. Invite family members to special occasions that are available to the residents.

3. Offer guidelines for the best type of involvement, such as the "do's" and "don'ts" in Alzheimer's disease.

4. Show interest and care for residents. Help family members to understand the situations that their loved ones experience. In a real way, the staff service is for family members, too.

Such suggestions can become a reality in long-term care when staff members have a firm understanding of how important it is to recognize the needs of family members and to find ways to accommodate those needs. Ways of implementing strategies that could potentially meet the family needs expressed in the previous suggestions are as follows:

•   Staff members should make it a priority to let family members know where they are during visits and should verbally express how important the family members' visits are to the residents. When families receive affirmation regarding the importance of their post-admission involvement, they may feel more compelled to continue to participate in the lives of their elderly relatives.

•   When it comes to family participation in activities, staff members can offer verbal invitations to upcoming events to family members upon their visits to the facility. Many facilities also have large calendars in several areas of the unit that display the upcoming activities so they are visible to residents and visitors. For those family members who do not visit regularly, sending invitations via conventional mail is a way to inform families about upcoming activities and to emphasize the importance of their presence at these activities.

•   Offering guidelines for the best type of involvement is one of the most important ways CNAs can help families continue their involvement. This includes educating families about the most effective approaches for staying involved in the lives of older relatives, especially those with AD. Many families are at a loss when their relative develops AD, and instead of staying involved, they tend to withdraw after experiencing negative incidents during visits. CNAs should familiarize families with typical behaviors that are sometimes displayed by individuals with AD (e.g., verbal aggression, agitation, aggressive behaviors) and educate them on ways to handle these behaviors through effective and appropriate communication strategies (e.g., VT and reality orientation). In addition, CNAs should teach families what not to do in difficult situations and assure them that staff members are always available to answer questions and provide assistance in any situation.

- Staff members should consider themselves allies to family members. CNAs must understand that their responsibilities extend beyond the care they provide for residents. Admitting a relative to a long-term care facility is a major transition in the lives of family members as well, and they, too, rely on staff in many ways. CNAs must therefore instill a sense of trust with family members through positive and reciprocal communication and should offer advice and feedback to families who want to remain active in the lives of their older relatives. Finally, CNAs must emphasize that families are a vital component of their relative's care and well-being and that their continued involvement will always be necessary.

The testimony of a wife who has continued her involvement in the life of her husband, who has had AD for more than a decade, illustrates the importance of continued involvement for family members.

We [my husband and I] have embarked on a long, long journey. It is not a journey we chose to make, but rather a journey dealt to us by fate. Alzheimer's disease has played a major role in our lives for the past $12^1/2$ years. For the first 10 years after his diagnosis, my husband was at home with me, and for the past $2^1/2$ years he has been a resident at Chapel Hill Community.

In the beginning I went to see him three times a day, sometimes arriving before the 7:00 A.M. shift. At that time, my husband was mobile and fell quite frequently, so I spent much time there with him to monitor his activities and try to prevent falls. After he was confined to a wheelchair I went only twice a day, at noon and in the evening to feed him, as he could no longer do it himself. I usually arrived between 10:00 and 11:00 A.M. and waited until he was down for a nap around 1:00 or 1:30 P.M. Then I went home until 4:00 P.M. and came back in to feed him his supper, staying until about 6:00 P.M.

Mainly I go because I want to be there. However, I feel I am needed because I know he is comforted by my touch and my voice. Although my greatest responsibility is to my husband, of course I do feel a certain responsibility to his nurses and nursing assistants. Anything I can do to lighten their load I will do. It takes a certain kind of person to do this work and I thank them from the bottom of my heart for their patient consideration and the love they manifest daily as they care for our loved ones.

It is all worth any effort on my part when I see the occasional crinkle of his eyes or familiar smile on his face, even if just for a fleeting moment. Each time I leave, I leave part of me behind. Truly, Alzheimer's disease is a kaleidoscope of feelings and emotions, constantly in a state of change.

BARRIERS TO PROMOTING FAMILY INVOLVEMENT

Implementing strategies for increasing family involvement is an ideal notion for facilities and dedicated staff. However, potential barriers exist for CNAs within the long-term care system. CNAs, unfortunately, are faced with a variety of challenges that may interfere with their ability to help promote family involvement in long-term care. These barriers include inadequate CNA staffing, high rates of staff burnout, and feelings experienced by many CNAs of inferiority and disrespect.

In order for CNAs to provide successful and consistent interaction with family members, they must utilize time during their shifts to do so. This can be problematic, however, in that the majority of long-term care facilities are understaffed, causing difficult workloads for individuals to sustain. The shortage of nursing assistants in long-term care settings makes it increasingly difficult for CNAs to accomplish additional tasks distinct from their daily care routines, thus allowing them fewer opportunities to interact with family members. These difficulties are expressed in the words of CNAs themselves:

> It would be nice to have the extra time to associate with family members during the day, but sometimes I don't feel that I even have enough time to provide adequate care to my residents, let alone to their family members. Our unit is understaffed as it is, and there are call-offs almost every day. Between bathing, feeding, dressing, and all of my other duties, I don't have time to do anything extra.

> I love to see family members come in to see our residents. It is so good for the residents, and you can see how happy it makes them. Usually I only have time to say a quick hello to the families, and I have to keep going so I can finish all of my work on time. There just aren't enough of us on the floor to stop and communicate with families as often as we would like. There have been plenty of times when I wanted to stop and talk to a family member, but on an Alzheimer's unit, you have to constantly be watchful of what is going

on, especially if we are short staffed. Stopping to talk to families just isn't possible all of the time.

In addition to being understaffed and having limited time to accomplish tasks aside from direct, hands-on care, CNAs often experience high rates of burnout and fatigue as a result of their job demands. Burnout, especially for full-time staff members, can negatively affect job performance. When an individual experiences burnout as a result of job demands, he or she typically does not invest additional amounts of time and energy in tasks that are not associated with normal care routines. If staff members lack energy and motivation, then it is highly unlikely that extra effort will be placed into implementing family involvement strategies.

The ways that CNAs are treated in the facility will have an impact on how they contribute to the promotion of family involvement. If CNAs do not feel valued and respected at their job, very few will feel obligated to put forth the extra effort needed to promote family involvement. Sadly, CNAs are often viewed as uneducated and inferior to other staff members. Consequently, their input and suggestions are often overlooked and ignored by higher ranked staff. If CNAs are not receiving positive reinforcement for their input and work contributions, they may feel discouraged from trying to implement new family involvement strategies, as noted in this statement from a CNA working in a long-term care facility.

> Sometimes I feel like I'm at the bottom of the totem pole and nobody really appreciates how hard I work. Being a CNA is a lot harder than most people realize, and I don't feel that I get the respect and recognition that I deserve. If CNAs were respected and acknowledged for the amount of work they do in one day, I think you would see an improvement in the care and the attitudes.

Each of these barriers that CNAs experience must first be resolved if the process of implementing family involvement strategies is to be accomplished. It is evident that inadequate staffing is an obstacle in long-term care and ultimately affects the amount of time that CNAs can devote to increasing family involvement. In order to resolve staffing shortages, facilities must maintain adequate staff-to-patient ratios so that CNAs have the ability to provide sufficient care in an allotted amount of time and still have the opportunity to interact with family members. Thus, one CNA should have no more than approximately 7 or 8 residents to care for in one shift. This becomes especially important on AD and dementia units, where increased staff supervision is required. Additional staffing strategies may include increasing the staffing of activity assistants, who are able to provide extra supervision and meaningful activities for residents to participate in. Activity assistants can also be used to encourage families to participate in ongoing activities and to ensure that appealing activities are being provided for residents and their families. Finally, having on-call CNAs, which many facilities now incorporate into their staffing routines, is an excellent way to ensure adequate staffing on a daily basis.

Resolving staffing issues not only provides more time for CNAs to complete additional tasks such as family interaction but also reduces their workload, which may eventually decrease the levels of burnout and fatigue among CNAs. The degree of burnout that a CNA experiences will have an impact on the amount of effort that he or she is able to contribute toward the implementation of strategies that are necessary for enhancing family involvement.

Aside from staffing issues, long-term care facilities must ensure that CNAs receive the same amount of respect and recognition that any other staff member receives. Acknowledging the amount of work and talent that CNAs contribute to facilities is critical for reinforcing their efforts and ideas and for encouraging a continuation of the highest level of care possible. This is evident in the following statement from a CNA working on an AD unit.

> The unit coordinator of the Alzheimer's unit that I work on would throw monthly staff appreciation parties and would provide food and small gifts for the staff members who worked on her unit. She would also recommend us for employee of the month and constantly compliment us on our job performance. With her in charge of the unit, we all felt like we were a family, and each of us felt appreciated for being there. No one ever felt like they were above or below other staff members because we were all valued equally, and our input and suggestions were always taken into consideration. This always made me feel more motivated to work harder and to make the unit better for our residents and their families. Not every Alzheimer's unit is like this, but they should be.

Overcoming the potential barriers that exist for CNAs and other long-term care staff is imperative for making progress on strategies that need to be utilized in order to promote family involvement. Before postadmission involvement from families can be increased, the conditions within the facility that prevent CNAs from engaging with families must first be identified and resolved. Only then can CNAs and their facilities achieve a desired level of family involvement.

CONCLUSION

Understanding the ramifications of a variety of strategies that have the potential to promote and increase family involvement leads to the successful utilization of these strategies in long-term care facilities. It is apparent that a majority of families choose to stay involved in the lives of their older relatives, even after their admission to long-term care. Because the caregiving role of the primary caregiver transfers from a family member to a staff member following admission, it becomes beneficial for both parties to work together to enhance the involvement process and to ensure the satisfaction of each person involved. Because maintaining and encouraging family involvement is extremely important for the well-being of both the family members and the residents, ways in which to promote this involvement must continue to be recognized and applied.

REFERENCES

Alzheimer's Association. (2000). *Validation method offers significant benefits to people with Alzheimer's disease and their caregivers.* Alzheimer's Association article 00078. Retrieved September 26, 2003, from http://www.charitywire.com/charity3/00078.html

Annerstedt, L., Elmstahl, S., Ingvad, B., & Samuelsson, S.M. (2000). Family caregiving in dementia—an analysis of the caregiver's burden and the "breaking-point" when home care becomes inadequate. *Scandinavian Journal of Public Health, 28,* 23–31.

Bleathman, C., & Morton, I. (1992). Validation method: A review of its contribution to dementia care. *British Journal of Nursing, 14,* 866–868.

Cohen, E. (1999). *Alzheimer's disease: Prevention, intervention, and treatment.* Lincolnwood, IL: Keats Publishing Group.

Davis, L., & Buckwalter, K. (2001). Family caregiving after nursing home admission. *Journal of Mental Health and Aging, 7,* 361–379.

Day, C. (1997). Validation therapy: A review of the literature. *Journal of Gerontological Nursing, 23*(4), 29–34.

Dippel, R., & Hutton, J. (1988). *Caring for the Alzheimer patient: A practical guide.* Buffalo, NY: Prometheus Books.

Feil, N. (1984). Communicating with the confused elderly patient. *Geriatrics, 39*, 131–132.

Feil, N. (1992a). The validation helping techniques can be used in each of the four stages that occur with late-onset demented populations. *Geriatric Nursing, 3*, 129–133.

Feil, N. (1992b). *V/F Validation: The Feil method* (Rev. ed.). Cleveland, OH: Feil Productions.

Feil, N. (1993). *The validation breakthrough.* Baltimore: Health Professions Press.

Feil, N. (2003). *The validation breakthrough* (2nd ed.). Baltimore: Health Professions Press.

Gaugler, J., Leitsch, S., Zarit, S., & Pearlin, L. (2000). Caregiver involvement following institutionalization: Effects of preplacement stress. *Research on Aging, 22*, 337–359.

Hansson, O., Nelson, E., Carver, M., NeeSmith, D., Dowling, E., Fletcher, W., et al. (1990). Adult children with frail elderly parents: When to intervene? *Family Relations, 39*, 153–158.

Helfer, K. (1991). Everyday speech understanding by older listeners. *Journal of the Academy of Rehabilitative Audiology, 24*, 17–34.

Naleppa, M.J. (1996). Families and the institutionalized elderly: A review. *Journal of Gerontological Social Work, 27*, 87–111.

O'Donovan, S. (1996). A validation approach to severely demented clients. *Nursing Standard, 11*(13/14), 48–52.

Ostuni, E., & Santo-Pietro, M. (1991). *Getting through: Communication when someone you care for has Alzheimer's disease.* Vero Beach, FL: The Speech Bin.

Pinquart, M., & Sorensen, S. (2003a). Associations of stressors and uplifts of caregiving with caregiver burden and depressive mood: A meta-analysis. *Journals of Gerontology. Series B, Psychological Sciences and Social Sciences, 58*, P112–P128.

Pinquart, M., & Sorensen, S. (2003b). Differences between caregivers and noncaregivers in psychological health and physical health: A meta-analysis. *Psychology and Aging, 18*, 250–267.

Riddick, C., Cohen-Mansfield, J., Fleshner, E., & Kraft, G. (1992). Caregiver adaptations to having a relative with dementia admitted to a nursing home. *Journal of Gerontological Social Work, 19*, 51–76.

Silliman, R.A., & Sternberg, J. (1988). Family caregiving: Impact of patient functioning and underlying causes of dependency. *The Gerontologist, 28*, 377–382.

Small, J., Kemper, S., & Lyons, K. (1997). Sentence comprehension in Alzheimer's disease: Effects of grammatical complexity, speech rate, and repetition. *Psychology and Aging, 12*, 3–11.

Smythe, J., & Haworth, G. (1995). Memories are made of this. *Primary Health Care, 5*, 20–22.

Tickle, E.H., & Hull, K.V. (1995). Family members' roles in long-term care. *Medical-Surgical Nursing Journal, 4*, 300–304.

Toseland, R., Diehl, M., Freeman, K., Manzanares, T., Naleppa, M., & McCallion, P. (1997). The impact of validation group therapy on nursing home residents with dementia. *Journal of Applied Gerontology, 16*, 31–50.

Touzinsky, L. (1998). Validation therapy: Restoring communication between persons with Alzheimer's disease and their families. *American Journal of Alzheimer's Disease, 13,* 96–101.

Vitaliano, P., Zhang, J., & Scanlan, J. (2003). Is caregiving hazardous to one's physical health? A meta-analysis. *Psychological Bulletin, 129,* 946–972.

Woodrow, P. (1998). Interventions for confusion and dementia. 4: Alternative approaches. *British Journal of Nursing, 7,* 1247–1250.

RESOURCES

Katherina A. Nikzad, B.A., is a certified nursing assistant in Ohio. She is pursuing her master's degree in social work as well as a doctorate in gerontology at the University of Kentucky. For more information and recommendations regarding the promotion of family involvement at the CNA level, please contact

Katherina A. Nikzad, B.A.
Graduate Center for Gerontology
The University of Kentucky
306 Health Sciences Building
900 S. Limestone
Lexington, KY 40536
E-mail: katherina.nikzad@uky.edu
Telephone: 330-284-4196
Fax: 859-323-5747

- For more information about the principles of Validation therapy, go to: http://www.vfvalidation.org/whatis.html ("What is Validation?")

- For books, articles, and videos on Validation therapy, go to: http://www.vfvalidation.org/articles.html ("Validation Resources") or http://healthpropress.com (Health Professions Press)

- For information on reality orientation, go to: http://www.zarcrom.com/users/alzheimers/t-02.html ("Reality Orientation")

4

Making the Long-Term Care Environment More Like Home

The Eden Alternative: What Families Want, and Why

JUDITH C. DREW

One of the biggest challenges facing researchers and gerontologists today is putting into practice the findings of studies that suggest how various types of living environments affect the quality of life and well-being of older adults. Although for decades several theorists, researchers, and practitioners have explored why and how person–environment interactions affect our quality of life, there is little agreement about how to design and manage habitats that best support the physical, psychological, and social well-being of older adults (Christenson & Taira, 1990; Gordon, 1981; Kahana, 1982; Lawton, Byerts, & Windley, 1982; Scheidt & Windley, 1998, 2003; Taira & Carlson, 2000; Wahl, Scheidt, & Windley, 2003; Ward, Sherman, & LaGory, 1988). The habitat of primary concern in this chapter is the nursing home, which residents and family members describe as having few attributes of a real home. In this chapter, an overview of concerns about the traditional nursing home environment is presented along with a brief description of The Eden Alternative as a philosophy capable of transforming institutional settings into enlivened environments that are more like home. Finally, thematic findings are reported from a qualitative study of family satisfaction with an Eden Alternative nursing home.

THE TRADITIONAL NURSING HOME ENVIRONMENT

Traditional nursing homes that look and feel like institutions continue to dominate the landscape of long-term care facilities, where approximately 5% of the elderly American population of Medicare recipients resides (Shankroff, Feuerberg, & Mortimer, 2000). Nursing homes in the United States are viewed as places where people go to die rather than to live stimulating and satisfying lives (Goffman, 1961; Kane, Kane, & Ladd, 1998; Rowles, Concotelli, & High, 1996). This reputation evolved over time from the experiences, perceptions, and realities of residents and family members who live in, provide care at, and visit these institutions. In addition to unfavorable reports from residents and families, researchers have discovered that, among older adults in residential care, a phenomenon called *failure to thrive* occurs (Egbert, 1996; Newbern & Krowchuk, 1994; Osato, Stone, Phillips, & Winne, 1993; Sarkisian & Lachs, 1996). Like the same-named phenomenon found among infants, manifestations of failure to thrive in the elderly population include poor nutritional status, frailty, decreased cognitive functioning, withdrawal from social interactions, depression, and the loss of independence, dignity, and control (Schultz & Williamson, 1993; Siegal, 1993). Many researchers associate this failure to thrive with the dull, cold, and standardized environment of some nursing homes that summarily strips individuals of their uniqueness and withholds the warmth and stimulation of a true home where souls are nourished and human development is nurtured (Carstensen & Erikson, 1986; Drew & Brooke, 1999; Hendy, 1987; Thomas, 1996).

Donnenwerth and Petersen (1992) reported that low levels of well-being among some nursing home residents are related to the pressures imposed by staff for them to adopt sick role behaviors rather than remain independent and in control of their daily lives. One factor cited in the literature as contributing to learned helplessness, depression, and loss of dignity is the staff's insistence that residents use wheelchairs to get around the facility rather than ambulate under their own power (Smithers, 1992). Practices such as these have been allowed to continue because they make the work of the staff predictable and less costly. Although standardized rather than individualized care is less costly for the organization, it contributes to poor health outcomes and decreased quality of life among residents (Jacelon, 1995; Shield, 1990). Despite evidence that institutions with more homelike environments encourage independence and produce more opportunities for improved quality of life among their residents, issues of cost, maintenance, and industry regulation remain barriers to basic cultural change in nursing homes.

ENLIVENED ENVIRONMENTS AS HOMELIKE SETTINGS

For decades, researchers and practitioners alike have proclaimed that traditional nursing home environments in no way resemble home (Carboni, 1990; Drew & Brooke, 1999; Lawton, 1976; Lawton & Cohen, 1981; Moos & Lemke, 1980; Pearson, Hocking, Mott, & Riggs, 1993; Smithers, 1992; Stirling & Reid, 1992). According to Carboni (1990, p. 32), "home is the experience of a fluid and dynamic intimate relationship between the individual and the environment (physical, social and psychological spaces)" where interactions between the two contribute significantly to the individual's identity, connectedness, autonomy, power, and meaning of life. Residents and families also recognize that nursing homes are not homelike in appearance, design, function, or milieu. Although some facilities are redesigning their interiors, brightening their façades, or filling voids in human companionship with birds, fish, and kittens, the fact remains that unless philosophical and cultural changes are made in how care is provided, no significant changes in the quality of life of nursing home residents will occur.

Although redesigning an old building may not be economically feasible for most nursing home owners, there are models of enlivened habitats that can philosophically, culturally, and functionally transform a traditionally stark and lifeless nursing home into a warm and nourishing homelike setting. By definition, homelike settings include more than superficial decorations and familiar furnishings. Koncelik (1976) suggested that a true sense of home requires the personalization of all living spaces so that social interaction is stimulated, meaningful activities are encouraged, and each person expresses some measure of control over how space is used. In addition, maximizing the safety, function, and independence of all residents at all levels of cognitive and physical ability is facilitated when the environment is filled with familiar cues such as pleasant memories, loving pets, plants that need care, and visiting children. The preservation of human dignity and an overall quality of life are dependent on the nursing home resident's ability to navigate the environment safely, freely, and independently (Trabert, 1996).

The significance of a true homelike, enlivened nursing home environment filled with pets, plants, and visiting children is that it provides residents with multiple opportunities for companionship, independent functioning, dignity, and control (Barba, Tesh, & Courts, 2002). According to Dr. William H. Thomas, creator of The Eden Alternative, enlivened environments in nursing homes reduce the boredom, help-lessness, and loneliness among residents when the care provided is guided by a social model rather than a medical model (Thomas, 1996). A social model of care views caregiving as a reciprocal act whereby both the givers and receivers experience pleasure, pride, and a sense of accomplishment. In contrast, although incredibly important to health and quality of life, the medical model bases its approach on the principle that a dominant party gives care to promote a cure in a dependent person through the use of prescribed treatments. With regard to applying a social model to the development of enlivened environments, Carboni (1990) has reminded us of the social nature of human beings and the necessity of interaction between them. She demanded that our philosophies of care, environmental designs, and daily operations foster reciprocal relationships and a sense of belonging while preserving the individual identities of persons residing within the larger commu-nity.

Major decisions about changing approaches to care away from the medical model and toward a social model must start at the top of the organization and include staff at all levels, family members, and the residents themselves. Corporate philosophies and missions, boards of directors, administrators, and managers all must support the transfor-mation to an enlivened, homelike environment and provide the educa-tion and resources to sustain such a change (Moore, 1999). Education and involvement in planning, maintenance, and evaluation must also traverse all levels of staff, include family members, and involve the community at large. The organizational climate must welcome and value the participation of all constituents in order to make an enlivened environment a lasting reality. Although several models of enlivened environments have been proposed, The Eden Alternative has been most successful in helping to guide changes in nursing home culture (Sloane, Zimmerman, Gruber-Baldini, & Barba, 2002).

RECENT TRENDS IN CULTURAL CHANGE

The Eden Alternative is the most popular modern philosophy used to guide the transformation of traditional nursing home settings into full and thriving habitats for older adults (Thomas, 1994). Others have copied this prototype or watered down its approach, but The Eden

Alternative remains the most noted and complete cultural change in the nursing home industry. Thomas purported that this innovative approach to making nursing home environments look and feel more like home is capable of enhancing the general well-being of residents while reducing loneliness, boredom, and helplessness. Thomas's mission, *to improve the lives of elders and their caregivers by transforming the communities in which they live and work,* is built upon three fundamental premises about human growth for nursing home residents, staff, and potentially even family members. The first premise suggests that the potential for human growth is never lost among staff, residents, or family and that each person grows because of interaction, companionship, and reciprocal caring. The second premise establishes care as a selfless act, oriented toward helping others to grow. The third premise characterizes giving care and receiving care as continuous and lasting phenomena.

To facilitate the implementation of The Eden Alternative's mission and premises, Dr. Thomas and his associates offer workshops, recommend consultants, and provide supportive materials in a variety of different formats. One visit to The Eden Alternative web site (http://www.edenalt.com) provides interested parties with information about The Eden Alternative, including workshop dates and locations, newsletters, stories about nursing homes that have made the change, and resources that are available to assist nursing homes during and after the transition. Although Dr. Thomas stopped short of prescribing step-by-step, "how-to" instructions about implementing The Eden Alternative, he emphasized that this cultural change must be carefully planned and carried out over a relatively short period of time to maximize momentum and minimize resistance (Thomas, 1994). He also emphasized that successful implementation of The Eden Alternative is associated with having a clear set of goals and objectives, educational programs for all constituents, active and dedicated involvement by community members, resident-focused interventions, and unwavering commitment from owners, corporate executives, managers, and staff. Although a change of this magnitude is never easy, the story of one nursing home's journey to "Eden" is summarized in the following case example, as described by Drew and Brooke (1999), to inspire family members, their loved ones, and their caregivers.

In mid-1997, with strong support from corporate owners and the board of directors, a 168-bed, mixed-case nursing home in Texas began its transformation to The Eden Alternative. Staff, residents, and family members participated in education sessions, identified time and talents they could offer to The Eden Alternative, and pledged to work together to empower themselves. Creative teams of staff, residents, family members, and community volunteers worked to fill the environment with birds, cats, dogs, green plants, and children. Aviaries, fish tanks, and scratching posts soon became gathering places and topics of discussion for residents, who had previously sat silently in their wheelchairs without opportunities for reciprocal caring and interaction. Each day, donations of fresh flowers, pet food, animal care services, and artistic performances poured in from the community. The children's care center across the street from the facility brought the children to visit residents every afternoon. Some residents took turns reading aloud to the children while others provided warm laps and hugs. The laughter of the children and their warm smiles and soft touches brought back memories of what life was like *at home* for residents and family members alike.

COSTS VERSUS BENEFITS: THE RISKS OF CHANGE

Although The Eden Alternative gives residents and families new hope for improved quality of life, owners and operators of nursing homes express concerns about capturing and covering the costs of sustaining The Eden Alternative. First, costs associated with implementing and sustaining enlivened habitats are difficult to capture. Some facilities, for example, receive generous subsidies of their programs by community constituents such as florists, veterinarians, pet shops, child care agencies, schools, Boy Scouts and Girl Scouts, and volunteers who assist with training and servicing the pets and plants. In addition, dedicated gifts received from families and friends contribute to reducing the initial outlay of expenses associated with putting The Eden Alternative into place. Finally, several facilities throughout the United States and Canada have earned grants from local, state, and national foundations to support their Eden initiatives and research programs, making cost estimates more complex. Therefore, it is a challenge for facilities trying to make a decision to adopt The Eden Alternative to identify and plan for related costs that must be worked into an operating budget, given the diverse community and financial resources various nursing home settings have at their disposal.

In addition to concerns about costs, facilities as well as clinicians express worry about allergies some residents might have to animals, how residents will react to the death of their pets, and how the regulators in each state will view the building and organizational plans that facilities develop to control for increased hygiene and sanitation needs. Since the inception of The Eden Alternative, the scientific community has been critical of the small number of research studies conducted to examine claims about the difference that The Eden Alternative makes in the lives of nursing home residents. Researchers agree that systematically conducted research programs that analyze outcomes associated with The Eden Alternative must be performed in greater numbers to provide reliable evidence that this approach is responsible for improving the quality of life of nursing home residents and thereby to convince owners to spend money to change nursing homes.

FAMILY PARTICIPATION IN EDEN ALTERNATIVE PROGRAMMING AND RESEARCH: VOICES FOR RESIDENTS

Perhaps the most outspoken and important members of the nursing home community are the families who advocate for their relatives who live there. The voices and actions of family members have long been reported by investigators as important to setting standards of care and promoting well-being among nursing home residents (Bauer & Nay, 2003; Gaugler, Anderson, Zarit, & Pearlin, 2004). According to Hertzberg, Eckman, and Axelsson (2003), nurses in long-term care settings describe family members as important to the security, safety, and psychosocial well-being of the residents. Nurses noted the critical roles family members play in monitoring the environment and expressing specific ideas about what should happen there. For example, family members told Morgan and Stewart (1999) that they expect the modern-day nursing home to provide a safe, homelike environment, filled with stimulating activities and multiple opportunities for social interaction as well as privacy. These findings and many others reported in the literature (e.g., Bowers, 1988; Friedemann, Montgomery, Rice, & Farrell, 1999; Ryan & Scullion, 2000) provide evidence to support the inclusion of family members in planning, implementing, and evaluating The Eden Alternative.

In the late 1990s, families of the residents living at one of the nursing homes in southeast Texas were among the first to be consulted when a decision to adopt The Eden Alternative was being considered.

With grant funding from the Moody Foundation, the nursing home, its families, and its research partners at the University of Texas Medical Branch School of Nursing and Sealy Center on Aging joined forces to implement, sustain, and evaluate the cultural change. Family members were enthusiastic yet understandably skeptical about keeping pets and live plants in the facility. Fears focused on potential threats to safety and health. However, concerns were quickly put to rest as soon as care plans for each sector of The Eden Alternative community were put into place (Hendy, 1987). Family members spent many hours discussing with staff and researchers the changes they expected The Eden Alternative to make and which outcome variables they wanted measured in each cohort. After several meetings and educational sessions, the longitudinal evaluation research plan was designed and institutional review board approval was granted. Over the next 2 years, data were gathered at specific intervals using a series of questionnaires and interviews with nursing home staff, eligible residents, family members, and visiting children. Consent was obtained from each participant. Only the research findings from the sample of family members are included in this chapter.

Data Collection and Sample Demographics

Survey and qualitative data were collected from the sample of family members at 12 months after the implementation of The Eden Alternative (time 1) and again at 24 months (time 2) after the implementation. The instrument used to collect data from family members in this study was the Family Satisfaction Questionnaire for Nursing Homes (FSQNH; Vital Research, Inc., 1997). Initially developed as a tool to help nursing homes benchmark their performances and market their services, the survey was used here to determine if and how family satisfaction with the nursing home changed over time and during exposure to The Eden Alternative. To accomplish this, a total of 154 surveys and cover letters were mailed to the addresses of family members and residents' agents or guardians. Recipients were instructed to complete and return the survey to the researchers by postage-paid mail or by dropping it into a designated box at the facility. Reminder cards were sent out to all addressees 5 weeks after the initial mailing of the survey questionnaire.

Forty-one percent of the mailed surveys were returned at time 1 and 52% at time 2. The sample of respondents predominantly comprised women (time 1 = 54%; time 2 = 59%) who were children of the residents (time 1 = 45%; time 2 = 75%) and who ranged in age from 45 to 64 years (time 1 = 43%; time 2 = 60%). The most frequently occurring visiting pattern among the sample was 1–6 times per week (time 1 = 69%; time 2 = 78%), with 32% (time 1) and 41% (time 2) of respondents reporting that they actively participate in the care of their relative during each visit to the nursing home.

The survey items in the forced-choice portion of the FSQNH (Vital Research, Inc., 1997) asked respondents to indicate their opinions about communication patterns in the nursing home, the degree of resident autonomy and freedom they observed, the types of companionship provided, and the staff's responsiveness to the residents' requests for assistance. Family members were also asked to rate the environment, food, safety, their experiences with problem resolution, and if they would recommend this nursing home to others and why.

Statistical Analysis

Although there are no statistically significant changes in levels of satisfaction to report between time 1 and time 2, the ratings for communication, autonomy and freedom, and general responsiveness of staff to resident requests for assistance all increased over time and remained above the national benchmarking standard. It is also important to note that reasons family members gave for recommending this nursing home to others were the friendliness of the staff, the cleanliness of the facility, the variety of activities it offered, and the open style of communication between families and staff members. Table 4.1 provides a sample of survey items from the FSQNH administered at 12 months and 24 months after The Eden Alternative was implemented.

Themes in Family Narratives

In addition to responding to the categories of survey items described previously, family members were asked to write out responses to the following questions, which are the focus of the remaining report of findings included in this chapter.

Table 4.1. Percentages of family satisfaction with nursing home characteristics over time

Nursing home characteristics rated by family members	Benchmark satisfaction[a]	Actual percent satisfied, time 1 (12th month)	Actual percent satisfied, time 2 (24th month)
Resident interacts with other residents	77	98	99
Resident has voice in daily decisions	71	78	83
Staff is responsive to resident's needs	79	88	90
Staff is friendly	50	88	90
Environment is clean and odor free	88	93	97
Activities are available for all levels	72	85	94
Problems are resolved quickly	83	90	93
Overall satisfaction with the nursing home	82	91	91

[a]Data from Vital Research, Inc. (1997). *Resident experience and assessment of life: A resident and family satisfaction program for long-term care.* Los Angeles: Applied Evaluation Survey Research.

1. Why does your resident like the nursing home?

2. Why do you like the nursing home?

3. What could be done here to make things better for your resident?

The narrative responses given by family members at time 1 and time 2 were analyzed for emergent themes and are reported here in detail.

Why does your resident like the nursing home?

The dominant themes in the responses of family members to this question reveal their beliefs that residents are comforted by a *very helpful staff,* experience pleasure about the fact that there are *lots of things to do,* and enjoy the *love of all of the animals* living at the nursing home. Many family members who made comments on behalf of their relatives stated that the nursing assistants seemed genuinely interested in the residents, which made each resident feel cared for in a nice, friendly environment. One daughter commented that her mother always said, "she never knew kinder or nicer people to care for her and help her meet her needs." Another very satisfied daughter remarked, "This is home to [my father], and when we take him out for a holiday dinner he is in a rush to get back to all the animals and activities." Throughout the responses, family members repeatedly emphasized the positive influence many activities had on resident quality of life. These remarks are best summarized by a son who valued the fact that, although "many opportunities are available, they are not pushed on the residents" and a daughter who summed up her mother's thoughts when she said, "Mother enjoys being busy all day with something productive to do."

Although early in The Eden Alternative several families expressed concern over animals residing in the nursing home, the love and companionship the animals provided during interactions with the residents helped families to accept the positive differences they made. One of the blind and bed-bound residents had daily visits from a guinea pig that nuzzled up against her neck and wiggled its cold nose on her cheek. The smile on her face and the long strokes of returned loving touch said much more than words can describe. This resident's daughter explained that her "mother is an animal lover and the Eden program has helped her tremendously. She has experienced relief of her depression, and I think this program is extremely important." Even though family members were not prompted to qualitatively comment about specific aspects of the environment, one husband commented that his wife "thinks she is at home because of the animals, birds, and gardening." Finally, an emotional daughter told us that The Eden Alternative was responsible for her mother's well-being and that "it has really allowed her to use her talents and has encouraged her to re-develop talents she had not used in years. This has made her feel useful again."

Why do you like the nursing home?

In addition to representing the feelings of their relatives, family members were asked to tell researchers what they themselves liked about the nursing home. In their stories are themes that reveal their happiness about *a friendly staff with caring attitudes,* how important *the clean and attractive environment* is to them, and beliefs they have about what The Eden Alternative does to improve *the quality of activities and life* for the residents. Family members said, "I like that most of the staff is friendly and most of the employees are nice and courteous and helpful" and "The staff is good and friendly and really seems to care; there is a very caring group of aides here." Even though several family members suggested that they liked the nursing home because it was close to their work or house, convenience was secondary to their desires for a clean, attractive, and odor-free environment. "This nursing home is cleaner than most," said one daughter, and another daughter commented, "This nursing home also offers a secure and friendly environment for the most part."

Although the comments made seem rather generic when it comes to anticipating the responses family members might give when they are asked about what they want in a nursing home, The Eden Alternative was mentioned by name throughout the narrative comments. One family member said, "I particularly like the Edenization program. The activities staff has done a great job and I'm pleased with my mother's participation." Another commented, "The Eden Program is enjoyed by all—residents, staff, administration, families. The facility and the gardens are attractive and usually well kept and clean." Perhaps the influence of The Eden Alternative at this nursing home is best described by a daughter who said, "They have done a wonderful job of implementing Eden. There are happier, smiling faces found more and more frequently around here. There is definitely more life on campus."

For researchers and clinicians alike, qualitative findings such as those reported here have great practical significance even though statistical significance is difficult to establish, both in this study and other quantitative/empirical evaluations of The Eden Alternative. Seeming to address Dr. Thomas's claims specifically, one of the wives who participated in this research study remarked, "The Eden theme gives the residents a strong impression of self-worth . . . that someone cares enough for them to go to all the trouble."

What could be done here
to make things better for your resident?

Although the aim of The Eden Alternative evaluation research program was to discover changes in resident outcomes and family satisfaction over time, data were also collected to enhance the already rigorous continuous quality improvement program functioning in this nursing home. The dominant themes in the responses of family members to the question, "What could be done here to make things better for your resident?" revealed an overwhelming appeal for *more staff* and a desire for *better food service* and *improvements in laundry services*. Comments that provide support for these emergent themes include concerns expressed about too few staff, especially on the weekends; food served cold and too spicy; and lost clothing. Many family members agreed that, on any day of the week, "additional staff would help."

Understaffing is a well-known and common problem in nursing homes and one that is complicated by a high turnover rate among nursing assistants. For example, as research on nursing homes has consistently emphasized, turnover of nursing assistants and other staff members is considerable (in some studies, as high as 400%), and such disruption appears to influence outcomes ranging from hospitalization and infection on the part of residents to overall assessments of quality of care (Castle, 2001; Harrington & Swan, 2003). Although The Eden Alternative is designed to empower staff and support their needs for feeling valued and cared for, the short supply of long-term care workers plagues the entire industry and threatens the quality of care for a large number of nursing home residents. As the popularity of The Eden Alternative grows, there will be more and more opportunities for nursing home staff to find satisfaction in their work and reap the rewards of knowing that they help their older clients live full lives.

One of the resident's wives recommended a remedy for dissatisfaction with the food that is consistent with The Eden Alternative philosophy. She suggested, "perhaps the cooks can get some recipes from the residents or at least some ideas for specific dishes; perhaps old-fashioned favorites. This will make them feel at home . . . all the good smells and memories." This is certainly an idea that has the potential to contribute to a homelike environment filled with participation from all those who live there. No one family member had a miracle cure for laundry problems. Of course, whenever a procedure requires the centralized processing of individually owned items, as does community laundry, damage and loss are highly probable outcomes. As one daughter put it, "My only complaint is the laundry service. I have just resigned myself to the fact that my mother will not have certain garments. It is most frustrating and I think it could be resolved." At the completion of this research study, a team of residents, family members, and staff was busy working on an Eden-based solution to the laundry problem. In the true spirit of Eden, other teams pulled together to address issues about food and staffing.

CHALLENGES ASSOCIATED WITH EDEN ALTERNATIVE RESEARCH

As with any research project conducted in the context of long-term care (Mentes & Tripp-Reimer, 2002), this study was limited by high attrition rates among residents, high turnover rates among staff, and decreased family involvement over time. Also pertinent to this study, the aggressive quality improvement program the nursing home had been pursuing for many years prior to implementing The Eden Alternative may have confounded the influence The Eden Alternative could have on rates of infection, falls, incontinence, psychotropic medication and restraint use, and depression among the residents. This phenomenon is seen as a source of bias among Eden Alternative proponents, opponents, and researchers as well, yet it has some value in explaining why many Eden Alternative research programs report few statistically significant differences in selected resident outcomes when measured before and after Eden Alternative interventions are implemented. Many facilities that adopt The Eden Alternative have previously undertaken other efforts to improve their quality of care, and the choice to pursue The Eden Alternative is an extension of their ongoing commitment to these efforts.

Another challenge to this type of research is reluctance on the part of family members to honestly disclose the dislikes they and their relatives have, for fear of reprisal (Ryan & Scullion, 2000). Although family fears are not considered a problem in this study, they certainly have emerged as an important issue in other research efforts (Maas, Kelley, Park, & Specht, 2002).

More studies are needed that focus on outcomes that residents, staff, and families experience during exposure to enlivened habitats in long-term care. It is understood that the social and ethical phenomena operating in such settings do not permit researchers to withhold interventions from any members of the population. It is also understood that many measures of well-being are not sensitive to the responses that older adults have to changing life situations. Therefore, creative and robust studies must continue as changes in the cultures of long-term care settings evolve and flourish.

CONCLUSION

It is interesting to note that so many of the promises made by The Eden Alternative are discussed by family members in their comments about what they and their relatives like about this nursing home. Cleanliness, friendliness, helpful employees, and a homelike environment dominate the stories they tell. Although no family members use terms such as *traditional environments* versus *enlivened environments* when discussing their opinions, the terms *home* and *homelike* are heard frequently. Also of note is the freedom family members perceive as active participants in the nursing home community. Family members who speak out as voices for nursing home residents also carry their messages throughout the facility as well as into the larger community. They know what they want for their relatives and demonstrate each day that their participation in Eden is a vital ingredient for a "life worth living" (Thomas, 1996). It is readily apparent that The Eden Alternative gives family members the power to influence change in the long-term care industry. In short, family participation is key to initiating and sustaining cultural change in nursing homes.

Although there is agreement in the scientific community that few studies provide statistically significant evidence that The Eden Alternative improves the lives of nursing home residents (Hamilton & Tesh, 2002), families participating in the study reported in this chapter provide convincing testimony that it can make a difference. How much, when, and for how long are questions that do not seem important to nursing home residents living in the moment, living as though they are at home, and living as valued, contributing members of their community.

Readers are urged to stay aware of new developments in homelike settings for the long-term care industry. The Green House Project (http://thegreenhouseproject.com), a new model for long-term care in America, borrows heavily from The Eden Alternative and focuses primarily on improving the quality of life of the nation's elders. Settings in which this model is employed are group homes designed to blend easily into the community and its surroundings. For more information about The Eden Alternative and the Green House Project, readers can explore the resources listed at the end of this chapter.

REFERENCES

Barba, B., Tesh, A., & Courts, N. (2002). Promoting thriving in nursing homes: The Eden Alternative. *Journal of Gerontological Nursing, 28*(3), 7–13.

Bauer, M., & Nay, R. (2003). Family and staff partnerships in long-term care: A review of the literature. *Journal of Gerontological Nursing, 29*(10), 46–53.

Bowers, B. (1988). Family perceptions of care in a nursing home. *The Gerontologist, 28,* 361–368.

Carboni, J.T. (1990). Homelessness among the institutionalized elderly. *Journal of Gerontological Nursing, 16*(7), 32–37.

Carstensen, L.L., & Erikson, R.J. (1986). Enhancing the social environments of elderly nursing home residents: Are high rates of interaction enough? *Journal of Applied Behavior Analysis, 19,* 349–355.

Castle, N.G. (2001). Administrator turnover and quality of care in nursing homes. *The Gerontologist, 41,* 757–767.

Christenson, M.A., & Taira, E.D. (1990). *Aging in the designed environment.* New York: Haworth.

Donnenwerth, G.V., & Petersen, L.R. (1992). Institutionalization and well-being among the elderly. *Sociological Inquiry, 62,* 436–449.

Drew, J.C., & Brooke, V. (1999). Changing a legacy: The Eden Alternative nursing home. *Annals of Long-Term Care, 7,* 115–121.

Egbert, A.M. (1996). The dwindles: Failure to thrive in older patients. *Nutrition Reviews, 54,* S25–S30.

Friedemann, M.L., Montgomery, R.J., Rice, C., & Farrell, L. (1999). Family involvement in the nursing home. *Western Journal of Nursing Research, 21,* 549–567.

Gaugler, J.E., Anderson, K.A., Zarit, S.H., & Pearlin, L.I. (2004). Family involvement in nursing homes: Effects on stress and well-being. *Aging & Mental Health, 8,* 65–75.

Goffman, E. (1961). *Asylums: Essays on the social situation of mental patients and other inmates.* Garden City, NY: Doubleday.

Gordon, B.L. (1981). *Understanding and promoting the resources of aging people: A guide to care, proper environment, and well-being.* Ft. Lauderdale, FL: Exposition-Phoenix Press.

Hamilton, N., & Tesh, A.S. (2002). The North Carolina Eden Alternative Coalition: Facilitating environmental transformation. *Journal of Gerontological Nursing, 28*(3), 35–40.

Harrington, C., & Swan, J.H. (2003). Nursing home staffing, turnover, and case mix. *Medical Care Research and Review, 60,* 366–392.

Hendy, H.M. (1987). Effects of pet and/or people visits on nursing home residents. *International Journal of Aging and Human Development, 25,* 279–288.

Hertzberg, A., Ekman, S.L., & Axelsson, K. (2003). Relatives as a resource, but . . . : Registered nurses' views and experiences of relatives of residents in nursing homes. *Journal of Clinical Nursing, 12,* 431–441.

Jacelon, C.S. (1995). The effect of living in a nursing home on socialization in elderly people. *Journal of Advanced Nursing, 22,* 539–546.

Kahana, E. (1982). A congruence model of person–environment interaction. In M. Lawton, T. Byerts, & P. Windley (Eds.), *Aging and the environment: Theoretical approaches* (pp. 97–120). New York: Springer.

Kane, R.A., Kane, R.L., & Ladd, R.C. (1998). *The heart of long-term care.* New York: Oxford University Press.

Koncelik, J. (1976). *Designing the open nursing home.* Stroudsburg, PA: Dowden, Hutchinson, & Ross.

Lawton, M.P. (1976). The relative impact of congregate and traditional housing on elderly tenants. *The Gerontologist, 16,* 237–242.

Lawton, M.P., Byerts, T.O., & Windley, P.G. (Eds.). (1982). *Aging and the environment: Theoretical approaches.* New York: Springer.

Lawton, M.P., & Cohen, J. (1981). The generality of housing impact on the well-being of older people. *Journal of Gerontology, 36*, 233–243.

Maas, M.L., Kelley, L.S., Park, M., & Specht, J.P. (2002). Issues in conducting research in nursing homes. *Western Journal of Nursing Research, 24*, 373–389.

Mentes, J.C., & Tripp-Reimer, T. (2002). Barriers and facilitators in nursing home intervention research. *Western Journal of Nursing Research, 24*, 918–936.

Moore, K.D. (1999). Health and the environment: Are we as life care professionals "making the best of it"? *Qualitative Health Research, 9*, 61–64.

Moos, R.H., & Lemke, S. (1980). Assessing the physical and architectural features of sheltered care settings. *Journal of Gerontology, 35*, 571–583.

Morgan, D.G., & Stewart, N.J. (1999). The physical environment of special care units: Needs of residents with dementia from the perspective of staff and family caregivers. *Qualitative Health Research, 9*, 105–118.

Newbern, V.B., & Krowchuk, H.V. (1994). Failure to thrive in elderly people: A conceptual analysis. *Journal of Advanced Nursing, 19*, 840–849.

Osato, E.E., Stone, J.T., Phillips, S.L., & Winne, D.M. (1993). Clinical manifestations: Failure to thrive in the elderly. *Journal of Gerontological Nursing, 19*(8), 28–34.

Pearson, A., Hocking, S., Mott, S., & Riggs, A. (1993). Quality of care in nursing homes: From the resident's perspective. *Journal of Advanced Nursing, 18*(1), 18–24.

Rowles, G.D., Concotelli, J.A., & High, D.M. (1996). Community integration of a rural nursing home. *Journal of Applied Gerontology, 15*, 188–201.

Ryan, A.A., & Scullion, H.F. (2000). Family and staff perceptions of the role of families in nursing homes. *Journal of Advanced Nursing, 32*, 626–634.

Sarkisian, C.A., & Lachs, M.S. (1996). Failure to thrive in older adults. *Annals of Internal Medicine, 124*, 1072–1078.

Scheidt, R.J., & Windley, P.G. (Vol. Eds.). (1998). *Contribution to the study of aging series: Vol. 1. Environment and aging theory: A focus on housing*. Westport, CT: Greenwood Publishing Group.

Scheidt, R.J., & Windley, P.G. (Eds.). (2003). *Critical contributions of M. Powell Lawton to theory and practice*. New York: Haworth.

Schultz, R., & Williamson, G.M. (1993). Psychosocial and behavioral dimensions of physical frailty. *Journal of Gerontology, 48*, 39–43.

Shankroff, P.M., Feuerberg, M., & Mortimer, E. (2000). Nursing home initiative. *Health Care Financing Review, 22*(1), 113–115.

Shield, R.R. (1990). Liminality in an American nursing home. The endless transition. In J. Sokolovsky (Ed.), *The cultural context of aging: Worldwide perspectives* (pp. 331–353). New York: Bergin & Garvey.

Siegal, J.S. (1993). *A generation of change: A profile of America's older population.* New York: Russell Sage Foundation.

Sloane, P.D., Zimmerman, S., Gruber-Baldini, A.L., & Barba, B.E. (2002). Plants, animals, and children in long-term care: How common are they? Do they affect clinical outcomes? *Alzheimer's Care Quarterly, 3*(1), 12–18.

Smithers, J.A. (1992). A wheelchair society. In J.F. Gubrium & K. Chamaz (Eds.), *Aging, self, and community: A collection of readings* (pp. 237–255). Greenwich, CT: JAI Press.

Stirling, G., & Reid, D.W. (1992). The application of participatory control to facilitate patient well-being: An experimental study of nursing impact on geriatric patients. *Canadian Journal of Behavioural Science, 24,* 204–219.

Taira, E.D., & Carlson, J.L. (Eds.). (2000). *Designing, adapting, and enhancing the home environment.* New York: Haworth.

Thomas, W. (1994). *The Eden Alternative: Nature, hope and nursing homes.* Sherburne, NY: Eden Alternative Foundation.

Thomas, W.H. (1996). *Life worth living: How someone you love can still enjoy life in a nursing home. The Eden Alternative in action.* Acton, MA: VanderWyk & Burnham.

Trabert, M.L. (1996). Living in the moment: Support in the early stages of Alzheimer's disease. *Activities, Adaptation and Aging, 20*(4), 1–20.

Vital Research, Inc. (1997). *Resident experience and assessment of life: A resident and family satisfaction program for long-term care.* Los Angeles: Applied Evaluation Survey Research.

Wahl, H.W., Scheidt, R., & Windley, P. (2003). *Aging in context: Socio-physical environments.* New York: Springer.

Ward, R.Z., Sherman, S.R., & LaGory, M. (1988). *Environment for aging: Interpersonal, social, and spatial contexts.* Tuscaloosa: University of Alabama Press.

RESOURCES

For additional information about the Eden Alternative and its potential benefits for families, residents, staff, and facilities themselves, please contact

Judith C. Drew, Ph.D., RN
Professor, The Joseph B. and Mary Alice Collerain Professorship
Fellow, Sealy Center on Aging
University of Texas Medical Branch
301 University Boulevard, Route 1029
Galveston, TX 77555
E-mail: jdrew@utmb.edu
Telephone: 409-772-8227
Fax: 409-747-1550

In addition, readers are invited to

• Learn more about The Eden Alternative at www.edenalt.com

• Enjoy the "Online News Hour: A Nursing Home Alternative" at www.pbs.org/newshour/bb/health/jan-june02/eden_2-27.html

• Read "The Eden Alternative to Nursing Home Care: More Than Just Birds" by Paul R. Willging at www.asaging.org/at/at-214/eden.html

- Read about "An Eden Alternative Community in Action" at www.eldercarealliance.org/eden_alternative

- See the "Dog Owners Guide: Eden Alternative" at www.canis major.com/dog/llanfair.html

II

Group- and Family-Based Strategies

5

Support for Families
in the Nursing Home Environment

Family Caregiving, Social Support,
and Support Group Benefits of The Family Project

TERRY PEAK

It is well known that unpaid, devoted family members provide the
most caregiving to relatives in long-term care. It is also well known that
the demands of caregiving can overburden family caregivers, endanger
their physical and emotional well-being, and affect their willingness to
continue to give care (Horowitz, 1985; Zarit, 1990). Social support
reduces many of the stresses associated with caregiving, improves
morale and life satisfaction, and enhances feelings of self-confidence
and self-esteem (Biegel, Sales, & Schulz, 1991; Cohen & Syme, 1985;
Wilson, Moore, Rubin, & Bartels, 1990). Although it is common for
caregivers to experience stress when they do not understand or cannot
manage the care recipient's behavior, feel isolated, or feel unsupported
(Zarit, Orr, & Zarit, 1985), caregiver *subjective perception* of the situation
may be the real key to calibrating the experience of stress (Pearlin,
Turner, & Semple, 1989). Social support, especially in a support group
setting, can reduce the *perceived* valuation of the stressor by directly
influencing how the stressor is evaluated (Cohen & Syme, 1985).

This chapter describes in detail a support group intervention for
family members of relatives in long-term care facilities and how such

The author would like to express appreciation to the Sunshine Terrace Foundation;
to her two student assistants, Michelle Maughan and Virginia Quinn; and to The Family
Project participants. A Utah State University Faculty Research Grant supported the Family Project.

a strategy is potentially beneficial for families dealing with the admission of a relative to a nursing home.

THE BENEFITS OF SUPPORT
GROUPS FOR FAMILY CAREGIVERS

Information, training, and education provided in a comfortable setting have been shown to positively influence caregivers' perceptions of stress by illustrating and reinforcing ways that their behavior change can result in more effective strategies for managing stressful care situations (Light & Lebowitz, 1989; Peak, 1993; Peak, Toseland, & Banks, 1995). Many participants find the social support available in a group environment to be effective at preventing care demands from overwhelming their coping abilities. The range of benefits includes 1) reduction in feelings of isolation, 2) the opportunity to share ideas and personal experiences in a supportive environment, 3) positive affirmation of the importance of the caregiving role, 4) the opportunity to share effective problem-solving and coping strategies, and 5) a temporary sense of respite from the burdens of caregiving (Barusch & Peak, 1997; Toseland, 1990).

Experiential similarity, a hallmark of support groups, appears to enhance empathic understanding and helps to normalize the caregiving situation. When everyone in the room speaks the same language and has similar real-life experience, a sense of ease is attained that would take much longer to achieve in any other type of group setting. Also, advice is more welcome when the participant who offers it is attempting to cope with similar situations (Pillemer & Suitor, 1996).

Support groups can provide more concrete benefits than enhanced feelings of comfort and well-being. For example, previous research on supports for family caregivers (Peak, 1993; Peak et al., 1995) demonstrated positive effects for care recipients in poor health when the *caregiver* participated in a support group. In that instance, beyond the positive subjective responses from participants (Labrecque, Peak, & Toseland, 1992), the support group intervention for spouse-caregivers also resulted in considerable health cost savings for the care recipients—on average, a savings of $7,600 per recipient. More surprisingly, those in the poorest health obtained the greatest savings—an average savings of $10,300 (Peak, 1993). In summary, support groups for families who must care for frail relatives appear to exert a wide range of benefits to participants and are a potentially cost-effective intervention for overburdened caregivers.

CONTINUING FAMILY
CAREGIVING INTO THE NURSING HOME

Family caregiving in the community constitutes a major emphasis of the gerontological research literature (e.g., Pinquart & Sorensen, 2003a, 2003b; Vitaliano, Zhang, & Scanlon, 2003). This focus, however, is most often on *at-home* care situations, and the implications for family caregivers upon admission of the care recipient to a nursing home have received far less attention. In part because of the emphasis on service delivery to family caregivers *in the community,* and the continuing belief that family care ends after admission, few established supports assist family caregivers with their adaptation to the nursing home setting. The support that is available is often targeted to family caregivers in the community, generally with the goal of bolstering families' efforts to prevent or delay expensive residential care.

To many, admission of a relative to a long-term care facility is considered the termination of caregiving responsibilities; in actuality, family involvement does not stop at the nursing home door (Bowers, 1988; Hansen, Patterson, & Wilson, 1988). The physical burdens related to the provision of direct, hands-on care assistance may decrease somewhat, but emotional ties continue. Family caregivers often visit residents in nursing homes and assist with hands-on care (Zarit & Whitlatch, 1992). They do not want to relinquish total responsibility for their relatives. Some caregivers consider placement simply one phase of a dynamic process that begins with the initial assumption of responsibility and ends with death (Pearlin, 1992). For example, the time pressure of maintaining visiting schedules, the perceived need to provide assistance and oversee care, financial issues, and residual guilt mean that caregiving stress may not decrease at all after admission (Friedemann, Montgomery, & Rice, 1999). In fact, a new stressor may emerge—the perceived ambiguity about the appropriate role for the family member in the nursing home environment when ensuring that appropriate care is provided to the resident (e.g., Rubin & Shut-tlesworth, 1983; Schwarz & Vogel, 1990; Shuttlesworth, Rubin, & Duffy, 1982).

To help maintain their involvement, families want relationships with staff who care for their relatives; for the caregiver, this is defined as high-quality care (Bowers, 1988; Duncan & Morgan, 1994; Tobin, 1993). Following admission, family members look for "ways to continue functioning as a family" (Friedemann et al., 1999, p. 19). They appreciate individualized interactions with nursing home staff, especially if that interaction acknowledges the unique, personal qualities of the resident (Friedemann et al., 1999). For example, if a staff member takes the time to mention an activity in which the resident participated, family members may perceive this as recognition of the resident as a person, rather than as just another task object.

This desire for the resident to be viewed as more than a task object warrants more scrutiny. Several researchers have questioned empirical analyses of caregiving in the nursing home that explore division of tasks. Using qualitative methods, these studies demonstrate that family members of older adults in residential care do not discuss caregiving in terms of task allocation but instead describe care by its purpose. For example, through in-depth, open-ended interviews with 28 caregivers, Bowers (1988) found that family members' primary purpose in remaining involved in the nursing home was to preserve the identity of the resident. Respondents identified different types of *preservative care,* such as maintaining family connectedness, ensuring the resident's dignity, helping the resident maintain control over his or her environment, and maintaining the resident's hopes. With the exception of family connectedness (e.g., bringing personal belongings to the resident), caregivers stressed that preserving the identity of the resident could be accomplished only through collaboration with nursing home staff. Often, family members felt it would be more effective in the long run to teach staff the way sensitive, nurturing, and individualized care should be provided rather than provide direct care themselves. Their expectation would be that aides and nurses would then deliver such care to the resident when the family members were not present. For example, caregivers in this study would tell staff stories that personal-ized the resident. They shared the affective/emotional outcome of pro-viding inadequate care and demonstrated effective care strategies to staff members. In instances in which caregivers could not observe spe-cific tasks being carried out, family members would "gather evidence" by monitoring the care provided to other residents. They asked the resident about the care provided (when possible) or tried to assess evidence of the emotional or psychological impact of staff care on the resident (e.g., depression, hopelessness, discomfort).

Additional qualitative research has reported similar findings. For example, Duncan and Morgan (1994) conducted focus group interviews with 179 family members who cared for residents in a nursing home. Family members relinquished almost all "technical" care (e.g., bed and body work) to staff and were not interested in increasing the number or range of tasks that *they* performed for their relatives. However, families did expect that staff would recognize them as vital informational resources who could provide insight that went far beyond the technical skills held by the staff. If staff members took advantage of this information, family members felt that the social and emotional aspects of care would be improved and would complement the technical assistance directed toward their relatives. Families were not only concerned with care *for* their relatives but also caring *about* their relatives (Duncan & Morgan, 1994). Families felt that quality care in the nursing home depended on staff treatment of the resident as a person, not as a task object, and on staff recognition that family involvement helped preserve the identity of the older adult (see also Hasselkus, 1988; Kellett, 1999; Rowles & High, 1996; Tilse, 1997).

Similarly, in a 3-year anthropological study of family involvement and decision making in four Kentucky nursing homes (Rowles & High, 1996; Rowles, Concotelli, & High, 1996), family members of residents were asked how much they felt they were involved in care-related decisions. Of the 229 family member contacts interviewed, almost half reported they were "fully involved" in care decisions related to crisis and life-and-death situations, competence of the resident, transfer of the resident, major financial needs, treatment/medical care, the social and physical environment of the resident, and daily living decisions. Overall, data revealed extensive family involvement across a wide range of care-related decisions. As with prior qualitative research, much of this involvement is related to individualizing and personalizing the care of residents. Family members attempt to preserve their relative's quality of life and maintain his or her links to the past.

Although the qualitative design of these various efforts limits generalizability to all residents or nursing homes, the rich open-ended data suggest a more complex role for family members following admission than those offered in analyses that rely on task-based assessments alone. That complexity may contribute to some of the difficulties family members encounter in their efforts to encourage care staff to move away from task-based care and instead offer more preservative dimensions of assistance. In The Family Project, we (the author of this chapter and two student assistants) wanted to explore how best to facilitate the provision of preservative care. The project's development is based on the belief that all involved—family members, staff, and residents—would benefit from an emphasis on more personalized care.

THE FAMILY PROJECT

Design

Based on the demonstrated challenges of family members of older adults in residential care, as well as the author's personal experiences as a family caregiver, we designed an intervention that would address some of the gaps in support for family caregivers. The objective of The Family Project was to help family members with their adjustment to the nursing home environment. Because support groups are well recognized as an effective format in which the presence of others with similar experiences enhances emotional well-being and understanding of problematic situations, The Family Project utilized support groups to provide education, accurate information, a support structure, and a safe environment in which to practice visiting techniques.

We planned the 8-week program design based on the family caregiving, social support, and nursing home literature. Our expectation was that, after 8 weeks, family adjustment to the nursing home environment would be improved. Our assumption was that an education-focused support group for family members, conducted right in the nursing home, would result in more frequent and more enjoyable visits and would also have a positive effect on family adjustment to the nursing home environment.

Project staff consisted of a social work faculty member (the author) and two undergraduate social work students; none were affiliated with the nursing home. Because this was a research project, some expenses associated with the students and the evaluation process were incurred that would not exist for a facility that decided to implement something similar. For example, we paid the students a small stipend for their involvement and reimbursed them for mileage. There were copying and postage expenses for handouts and evaluations. The project director was reimbursed for mileage to conduct interviews with participants and for 1 month's salary. Other costs could potentially fall to facilities willing to implement The Family Project. For example, several outside guest speakers were given $50 gift certificates to a local restaurant, and the facility covered the cost of refreshments for support group sessions (a relatively minor expense).

The facility in which The Family Project was implemented is a nonprofit, 172-bed facility accredited by the Joint Commission on Accreditation of Healthcare Organizations (essential for Medicare/Medicaid reimbursement) and serving individuals with a range of needs in either an extended care component, a special needs unit for those with memory loss, or a short-term rehabilitation unit.

To begin the project, the facility administrator sent introduction and reminder letters to all responsible family members of newly admitted (fewer than 6 months) residents at a local long-term care facility (see Appendix). A notice that announced the meeting was put in the local newspaper, and fliers were placed in the facility. The original target group was family members of newly admitted residents because we hypothesized that their need for support would be greatest; however, it became apparent that duration of nursing home residence was not necessarily correlated with reduction in need for information (or support). When they perceived a need, facility social workers and nurses referred other family members to the information sessions. For example, if a family member had a question about how many showers a resident could have in 1 week, why a resident's food preferences were ignored, or why a resident had been moved again, facility staff handed the family member a project information flyer and suggested that the family member attend the support group (see Figure 5.1).

All interested potential participants were invited to their choice of one of two information sessions during which The Family Project was

---

THE FAMILY PROJECT

Our first support group meeting will be held Tuesday, April 8, at 3:30 P.M. in the Living Room at [facility name]. This first meeting will give you the opportunity to learn more about the potential benefits to you of The Family Project.

WHERE: Living Room at [facility name]
WHEN: Tuesday, April 8, at 3:30 P.M.

Figure 5.1.   A project information flyer.

explained and project staff (the author and two student assistants) were introduced. Project staff members explained that we all had extensive caregiving experience and described that experience. Project staff members wanted to establish that they, too, spoke the caregiving language and had grappled with similar life situations. Project staff members explained that their own insecurities had led to the idea of a group that would combine support and education. They described these insecurities and explained how, despite professional training, there was always a great deal of uncertainty surrounding visits to the nursing home. For example, what was the recommended interaction for a resident with dementia? Should you give food or water to any resident who asked for it? What was the recommended response to a resident who asked to be taken home? And what should staff do about the occasional resident who simply screams?

Project staff members shared that, on occasion, all of us—project staff members and potential participants—had experiences where we felt ill-informed and unsure. The potential participants discussed all the things that bothered them or brought up subjects about which they wanted more information. Typical requests were for advice about how to relate to other residents, guidelines regarding what behavior is permitted (or not) during a visit, explanations of the different types of medications, answers to nursing home procedural questions (e.g., can residents be bathed more often if that is their preference?), and explanations of Medicaid rules and regulations. We explained that we anticipated at least one 8-week education-support group and possibly more. (The number of groups depended on the number of respondents. We wanted to limit participation to between 8 and 10 members.) We discussed potential topics and explained that the list of topics would be modified by what participants wanted to learn. At the end of the meeting, to reinforce what was discussed, an information sheet (see Appendix) was distributed so potential participants could review it more carefully at home.

After the two information sessions, family members who wanted to participate in the support groups indicated their interest by letter or phone call to the project staff members, or by contacting a staff member at the nursing home. This contact was followed by a telephone call to family members to confirm their desire to participate and to set up a time for a visit from one of the project staff, who, during that visit, administered the pretest evaluation instrument (Entrance/Exit Interview; see Appendix) and tried to clarify a personal goal for each participant and what, if any, specific information needs each person might have. We decided to establish a personal goal for each of the group members to help them experience a measurable sense of accomplishment at the conclusion of the support group (Barusch, 1991).

The information needs requested by group participants at the entrance interviews included the following:

- Appropriate responses to residents' "strange" behaviors

- Administrative issues that affect residents (e.g., internal moves, bathing procedures)

- Medical terminology used in resident evaluation

- Medications

- Different kinds of dementia

- Financial issues

- Department of Veterans Affairs rules and regulations

- Medicaid rules and regulations

- Future expectations

- The continual nature of caregiving

- Guilt, grief, and mourning

- Behavior changes in residents

- Resident interaction with the outside community (e.g., outside medical care)

- Problematic medical treatment issues (e.g., dental work beyond that necessary for good eating, reliability of vision testing, identification of glasses/dentures)

- Attitudes of other family members

Implementation

The Family Project was implemented on three separate occasions over the course of 15 months (without the research/evaluation component, however, implementation would involve a series of 8-week sessions for as long as a facility had people interested in participating). The Family Project groups met for 8 weeks in structured sessions that lasted from $1^1/2$–2 hours each. Each session had a stated topic prepared in advance by one of the students, the project director, or a guest; time for sharing what had happened to everyone (and their loved ones) during the previous week; and refreshments.

Topics included information about the typical medications used with older adults, Medicaid/Medicare rules and regulations and financial issues in general, caregiver self-care and stress reduction, nursing home concerns, caregiver guilt, and grief and mourning connected to changes in residents. During sessions, participants and facilitators shared personal experiences and their expertise as well as information about 1) the aging process and how various diseases, especially dementia, affect "normal" aging; 2) family interactions with nursing home staff; 3) effective communication with nursing home residents; 4) appropriate activities for the resident's health condition; 5) how to structure the visit as a positive encounter for all involved; and 6) caregiver self-care issues, such as relaxation and stress reduction techniques. Sessions were facilitated by one of the social work students and the project director and supplemented by nursing home staff members and outside speakers. The outside speakers were a psychiatrist, who explained medications; a psychologist, who spoke about guilt; and a representative from Medicaid, who provided information on current Medicaid rules and regulations.

Despite the original intention to limit group participation to family members of newly admitted residents, in the end, support group membership was not limited to any specific diagnosis, relationship to resident, or duration of nursing home residence. Relaxing the original exclusion criteria allowed us to maximize participation. There were a total of 19 participants across all three groups. Most participants (13, or 68%) were female. The groups included six spouses, ten children, one parent, and two other relatives (nieces). The length of time involved in caregiving ranged from less than 1 year to more than 10 years. Two family members worked full-time, two had never worked, five worked part-time, and ten were retired. Thirteen residents had a primary diagnosis of dementia, four had physical disabilities, and two had mental illness. The length of time of residence in the nursing home ranged from recently admitted to just under 2 years.

Participants expressed both specific and general information needs during the initial interviews. An example of a general information request was, "I would like to understand more how to take care of my mom, how to deal with her dementia. I think I could benefit if I knew more what it was like and what I could expect." A specific information need might be a question about the mechanism of interaction with the Department of Veterans Affairs or a request for information about psychotropic medications. The curriculum tried to incorporate both needs. It acknowledged family members' desire to continue to share in the care of their relatives as well as their need for support through the admission process and beyond. The curriculum also allowed individualized attention to specific information needs.

In the support group meetings, project staff—occasionally supplemented with nursing home staff, outside experts, or both—supplied information, answered questions, and tried to familiarize family members with the routine procedures and day-to-day resident life in the facility. Those participants with a longer history with the facility found it comforting to hear that some questions simply did not have good answers. For example, a common question is, "What happens to laundry that disappears?" Group participants felt better after the laundry procedures, with all of the steps taken to prevent losing laundry items, were described in detail, even though all participants understood that missing laundry might never be found. This sharing of information was expected to have a beneficial impact on the resident as well as the family member because "when family anxieties are eased, [the family's] interactions with the patient are relaxed" (Weiner, Brok, & Snadowsky, 1987, p. 153). Also, when family anxiety is reduced, frequency of visits may increase and family connectedness is maintained (Bowers, 1988). This process then results in an enhanced sense of partnership between family members and staff and a more enjoyable visit with the resident.

Because we implemented the intervention at three different times, we were able to learn (and improve) from our mistakes. For example, relaxation as a separate session topic was not added until the third iteration, whereas understanding medications and financial issues were consistently popular and were included in each 8-week session. The third consistent topic was facility staff interaction with residents. This particular topic consisted of either complaints about treatment by individual staff members or reactions to confusing facility policies; such sentiments were likely to be expressed at every session. Another result of multiple implementations is that the project staff experimented with the scheduling in an attempt to be convenient for all potential participants. The staff tried Saturday mornings once and late afternoons during the week twice. Both of these options were fine for some people, but it was impossible to achieve convenience for every participant.

Again, based on the authors' experience, the topic of appropriate medications is covered best by a psychiatrist. The psychiatrist that the project staff recruited as a speaker was able to explain quite clearly which patient symptoms lead to which medication choices. Other speakers might be able to explain what the medication was supposed to do, but only the psychiatrist could explain why it was chosen in the first place. However, as helpful as they are, psychiatrists are often quite busy. The second most popular guest chosen by project staff, a psychologist, gave a brilliant discussion about caregiver guilt. Both these professionals were difficult to schedule because of limited availability and would be expensive if they were compensated appropriately for their time. Project staff did not have enough money to pay speakers but did send them $50 gift certificates to a local restaurant as a token of appreciation. Even so, a large pool of available speakers is needed; otherwise, a group can quickly run out of willing experts. If the groups are scheduled in the evening or on Saturday, volunteer speakers might be easier to find.

The first sessions always started with introductions. Participants introduced themselves and talked about their relative and that individual's diagnosis and length of time as a resident. Group participants were invariably supportive of each other during these discussions. There was often an exploration and explanation of the admission decision-making process. It is possible that the guilt of that decision takes a long time to dissipate. For example, one participant stated as her personal goal, "I guess if you could help me feel better about putting her here and help me feel that it was the right thing." At these first sessions, participants visibly appeared to be struggling over their admission decision, no matter how long ago it had occurred, and would mention all of the options they had tried before admitting their relative to the nursing home. It was important for them to talk about who had given them "permission" to move forward with the admission process (usually a physician or religious leader). One participant said, "The doctor took one look at me and said, 'I'll see that he gets in.' "

Participants also struggled with the change in status from loyal spouse or child to concerned visitor: "Could I have lasted longer as a caregiver at home?" asked one. They also wanted to learn more effective ways to act as caregivers in the facility. This information need was expressed in personal goals such as "I guess I'd like to have some things to make my visits more meaningful to my husband if I can."

Whereas the first sessions were quite similar, second session topics varied over the three iterations. One session included appropriate visit activities, another covered medications, and yet another session addressed financial issues. The choice depended on our interpretation of the urgency of group participants' need for a particular type of information. We covered the same topics (e.g., the aging process, medications, nursing home concerns, Medicare/Medicaid, financial issues, guilt, grief and mourning, and caregiver self-care) each of the three times we implemented the intervention, but not always in the same order or in quite the same way. For example, when addressing caregiver self-care on the third iteration, we incorporated relaxation separately from stress reduction. This session started with a review of how the week went for each participant and resident. A brief video of the relaxation technique was shown. The group practiced the technique and received a handout that described that technique and others. Participants then shared positive experiences that occurred during visits with their relatives, followed by general reminiscences about their relatives. It was very rewarding to see the group members leave that session relaxed, smiling, and talking easily with each other.

Evaluation

As a condition of participation, group members agreed to a pretest and posttest evaluation. Family members agreed to 1) rate their perception of the condition of their relative, 2) rate their attitude toward the relative at the beginning and end of the intervention, 3) rate the quality of their visits to the facility, and 4) establish an individual goal at the pretest interview that would later be used to evaluate each individual participant's success (Barusch, 1991; see Appendix for the Entrance/Exit Interview). Outcome variables included perception of change in the resident (perception of resident change rating), change in attitude toward the resident (open-ended question in family interview), attendance at the sessions (facilitator record of number of sessions attended), perception of visit to facility (visit rating), and self-evaluation of the personal goal (goal attainment rating).

At pretest, family members were asked questions about length of time of caregiving, length of time their relatives had been in the nursing home, their relatives' primary diagnoses, upsetting behaviors in residents, their desire to be more involved in their relatives' care, and their current attitudes toward their relatives. Family members were also asked about social support received from friends and relatives, for a global health rating for themselves and if their health had ever been a problem to them, about financial worries and occupational status, and for a global mood rating.

In the posttest interview, family members were asked about their perceptions of change in those variables: change in the behavior of their relative, change in attitude toward the relative, and change in feelings about the relative. Family members were again asked a personal global health question and whether their own health had ever been a problem for them, and for a global mood rating. They were asked about their feelings about being a nursing home visitor and for suggestions of how the visitation process could be improved. Family members were also asked to rate specific Family Project session components and indicate their willingness to participate in any future projects.

Specific group components that received the most positive ratings were those that dealt with financial issues, Medicare/Medicaid rules and regulations, suitable visiting activities, causes of dementia, and medications. A well-received component of the project involved one of the social work students who worked directly with the residents connected to family members in the group. The student visited each of the residents individually and experimented with an assortment of visit activities (e.g., Scrabble, manicures, guitar playing, singing, storytelling). At the next group meeting, her experiences with these visit activities were shared with group members. This was beneficial in two ways: the family members simply enjoyed the knowledge that a new "friend" visited their relative, and they benefited from learning and sharing concrete examples of new activities. Participants said things like, "I was really thrilled that she was going in and talking to Mom," and, "Just the process of hearing about how she goes in, I'd have to say I've wanted to [visit] more." Also, a participant noted, "I think it helped give us some ideas of things we could do, too."

The responses to one question on the posttest interview form that requested open-ended qualitative responses were very positive. For example, one participant stated

> I think I have a little more in-depth understanding of what she's going through because of the group. I really enjoyed the people that have come in and did the different lectures, they were really good. I guess every time I go down I understand a little more or it's a little easier for me to take. I don't think I have particularly changed my attitude in caring for her, but I think my understanding of how it affects me is better.

Group members reported feeling less guilt in connection with the nursing home placement process. One participant said, "I really don't feel that I have to be there at a certain time, that she's waiting for me. I worried about that before [being in the group]."

Although many family members still found it demanding to visit the nursing home, they reported that it was easier than before participation in the support group. One participant said

> As far as my husband, I think I probably understand his problems a little more; it's been very beneficial for me, talking about the problems and asking questions and finding out. I think it was a learning experience, some of us we didn't quite know what to expect. It's still really hard to visit, but easier than it was.

Group members felt they learned to relate to their relatives better (e.g., were able to understand their individual situations a little better). As one noted,

> I still get upset although I understand her condition a little more. I've heard other people saying that so-and-so does the same kind of thing and I guess it just makes it easier for me to take—to understand that she's not really doing this just to make me miserable.

Participants also mentioned that they were going to miss knowing the group was there for them: "I've enjoyed the association with other people. You know you realize you're not alone and others have got worse problems than you have."

It is interesting that, although many family members reported that the upsetting behaviors in their relatives had gotten worse or that there was, at best, no change, the number of family members who reported enjoyment of their visits to the nursing home actually doubled from pretest to posttest (significant at the .001 level). Also, the number of family members who reported no enjoyment of visits decreased substantially from pretest to posttest. Clearly, support group participants felt better about visits to the nursing home after the intervention than they did before, despite the fact that, in most cases, their relatives were in worse health.

Initially, family members had identified a personal goal they wanted to accomplish during the project. Goals varied considerably and included financial issues, feelings about placement, dealing with dementia, relaxation, more meaningful visits, and dealing with depression. After the groups ended, most participants (76%) felt that they had made tangible progress toward their goals. One participant said,

"I feel less guilty. I learned from every one of them [group sessions] and particularly the reinforcement that you're not alone in this, that we're all in the same boat."

DISCUSSION

Outcomes for Family Project Participants

At the conclusion of The Family Project, support group participants felt better about visits to the nursing home than they did before, despite the fact that, in most cases, their relatives were in worse shape. All of the qualitative responses were very positive:

> We've learned some ways to get her mind off her problems and, when we go [visit], we have helped her with some of the good things that she liked to do. You find that almost everyone has to deal with a similar situation.

Some participants felt they had learned to relate to their relatives better (e.g., were able to understand their individual situations a little better). For example, one said, "Knowing that it isn't my fault that she is there. I blamed myself in the beginning. I still do somewhat but not as much as I did before." Other participants simply felt better after participation, commenting that, "I did make progress and saw the reasons why some of it, some things, were happening. It helped me to understand maybe her condition," and, "I haven't changed a lot of what I've done, it's just, it's been nice to realize other people are in with it, too. I think I got a better understanding of it [dementia] and that's what I was after, so it was very helpful." Participants said they would miss the group meetings: "I've just had a whole world open up to me as far as knowing about the nursing home. I am going to miss the group. I really am."

The positive responses from participants to the social support provided by the group were both encouraging and expected. Participants typically enjoyed support group interactions. What is especially surprising about the positive tone of this feedback, though, is the nature of this setting, which has a strong religious community as its base. The community predominantly consists of members of the Church of Jesus Christ of Latter-Day Saints. A hallmark of this religion is the social support that church members provide to each other. Yet, despite that, family members needed more help than they received from the support typically provided by friends and neighbors. Even in this case, participants were able to benefit from the social support that family members in similar circumstances could offer, which obviously went beyond the support that participants received through other sources.

Implications for Practice

With the information provided and the opportunity to role-play new behaviors in a safe and supportive environment, family members were better equipped to recognize the needs and reactions of their relatives and to find effective ways to respond to issues surrounding nursing home placement. They learned to deal more effectively with their own needs and shared their personal experiences and expertise with group members. This type of education and support group that targets family members of residents, offered directly in a long-term care setting, is a way for a facility to communicate to family members that it cares. Because perception is vital to the valuation of the visit experience, any method by which a long-term care facility can have a positive impact on this perception is worth pursuing.

In fact, although The Family Project has ended, because of its success, we continue to offer informal family meetings on a monthly basis to those who wish to participate. For the informal version, conducted by the same social work faculty member in a volunteer capacity, family members are notified of the next meeting with both a mailed flyer and a follow-up phone call. The nursing home provides supper (the same meal that the residents eat, which is an opportunity for family members to sample the food), which enhances the social and sharing features of the meeting. Family members are asked about any specific concerns, and otherwise receive fairly general information related to nursing home placement issues. The information needs of family members are reasonably predictable, thus preparation does not overburden the volunteer group facilitator. The meetings have become informal mechanisms through which family members can express any lingering admission anxieties as well as a convenient forum in which to share any other concerns.

There are obviously many potential methods to include family members into the nursing home environment. Family members are genuinely interested in establishing a positive relationship with nursing home staff and in continuing their involvement with the care of their relatives. With modest effort, a facility is able to reap large benefits for family members, residents, and staff. In our experience, a short-term combination of information, education, and social support intervention can be successfully and easily implemented in a long-term care setting, and family members will benefit from it.

REFERENCES

Barusch, A.S. (1991). *Elder care: Family training and support.* Newbury Park, CA: Sage.

Barusch, A.S., & Peak, T. (1997). Support groups for older men: Building on strengths and facilitating relationships. In J. Kosberg & L. Kaye (Eds.), *Elderly men: Special problems and professional challenges* (pp. 262–278). New York: Springer.

Biegel, D., Sales, E., & Schulz, R. (1991). *Family caregiving in chronic illness.* Newbury Park, CA: Sage.

Bowers, B. (1988). Family perceptions of care in a nursing home. *The Gerontologist, 28,* 361–368.

Cohen, S., & Syme, S. (1985). Issues in the study and application of social support. In S. Cohen & S. Syme (Eds.), *Social support and health* (pp. 3–22). Orlando, FL: Academic.

Duncan, M., & Morgan, D. (1994). Sharing the caring: Family caregivers' views of their relationships with nursing home staff. *The Gerontologist, 34,* 235–244.

Friedemann, M., Montgomery, R., & Rice, C. (1999). Family involvement in the nursing home. *Western Journal of Nursing Research, 21*(4), 549–567.

Hansen, S., Patterson, M., & Wilson, R. (1988). Family involvement on a dementia unit: The Resident Enrichment and Activity Program. *The Gerontologist, 28,* 508–510.

Hasselkus, B.R. (1988). Meaning in family caregiving: Perspectives on caregiver/professional relationships. *The Gerontologist, 28,* 685–691.

Horowitz, A. (1985). Family caregiving to the frail elderly. In C. Eisdorfer, M. Lawton, & G. Maddox (Eds.), *Annual review of gerontology and geriatrics* (pp. 194–246). New York: Springer.

Kellett, U.M. (1999). Transition in care: Family carers' experience of nursing home placement. *Journal of Advanced Nursing, 29*(6), 1474–1481.

Labrecque, M., Peak, T., & Toseland, R. (1992). Long-term effectiveness of a group program for caregivers of frail elderly veterans. *American Journal of Orthopsychiatry, 52,* 575–588.

Light, E., & Lebowitz, B. (Eds.). (1989). *Alzheimer's disease treatment and family stress: Directions for research.* Rockville, MD: U.S. Department of Health and Human Services.

Peak, T. (1993). Impact of a social support program for spouse-caregivers on the health costs and utilization of frail elderly veterans. *Dissertation Abstracts International, 54*(04), 125. (UMI No. 9323726)

Peak, T., Toseland, R., & Banks, S. (1995). The impact of a spouse-caregiver support group on care recipient health care costs. *Journal of Aging and Health, 7*, 427–449.

Pearlin, L. (1992). The careers of caregivers. *The Gerontologist, 32*, 647.

Pearlin, L., Turner, H., & Semple, S. (1989). Coping and the mediation of caregiver stress. In E. Light & B. Lebowitz (Eds.), *Alzheimer's disease treatment and family stress: Directions for research* (pp. 198–217). Rockville, MD: U.S. Department of Health and Human Services.

Pillemer, K., & Suitor, J. (1996). "It takes one to help one": Effects of similar others on the well-being of caregivers. *Journals of Gerontology. Series B, Psychological Sciences and Social Sciences, 51*, S250–S257.

Pinquart, M., & Sorensen, S. (2003a). Associations of stressors and uplifts of caregiving with caregiver burden and depressive mood: A meta-analysis. *Journals of Gerontology. Series B, Psychological Sciences and Social Sciences, 58*, P112–P128.

Pinquart, M., & Sorensen, S. (2003b). Differences between caregivers and noncaregivers in psychological health and physical health: A meta-analysis. *Psychology and Aging, 18*, 250–267.

Rowles, G.D., Concotelli, J.A., & High, D.M. (1996). Community integration of a rural nursing home. *Journal of Applied Gerontology, 15*(2), 188–201.

Rowles, G.D., & High, D.M. (1996). Individualized care: Family roles in nursing home decision-making. *Journal of Gerontological Nursing, 22*(3), 20–25.

Rubin, A., & Shuttlesworth, G. (1983). Engaging families as support resources in nursing home care: Ambiguity in the subdivision of tasks. *The Gerontologist, 23*, 632–636.

Schwarz, A., & Vogel, M. (1990). Nursing home staff and residents' families role expectations. *The Gerontologist, 30*, 169–183.

Shuttlesworth, G., Rubin, A., & Duffy, M. (1982). Families versus institutions: Incongruent role expectations in the nursing home. *The Gerontologist, 22*, 200–208.

Tilse, C. (1997). She wouldn't dump me: The purpose and meaning of visiting a spouse in residential care. *Journal of Family Studies, 3*, 196–208.

Tobin, S. (1993). Fostering family involvement in institutional care. In G. Smith, E. Tobin, A. Robertson-Tchabo, & P. Powers (Eds.), *Enabling aging families: Directions for practice and policy*. Beverly Hills, CA: Sage.

Toseland, R. (1990). *Group work with older adults*. New York: New York University Press.

Vitaliano, P., Zhang, J., & Scanlan, J. (2003). Is caregiving hazardous to one's physical health? A meta-analysis. *Psychological Bulletin, 129*, 946–972.

Weiner, M., Brok, A., & Snadowsky, A. (1987). *Working with the aged* (2nd ed.). Norwalk, CT: Appleton-Century-Crofts.

Wilson, P., Moore, S., Rubin, D., & Bartels, P. (1990). Informal caregivers of the chronically ill and their social support: A pilot study. *Journal of Gerontological Social Work, 15*, 155–170.

Zarit, S.H. (1990). Interventions with frail elders and their families: Are they effective and why? In M. Stephens, J. Crowther, S. Hobfall, & D. Tennenbaum (Eds.), *Stress and coping in late life families* (pp. 241–265). Washington, DC: Hemisphere.

Zarit, S.H., Orr, N., & Zarit, J. (1985). Interventions for families of dementia patients: A stress-management model. In S. Zarit, N. Orr, & J. Zarit (Eds.), *The hidden victims of Alzheimer's disease: Families under stress* (pp. 87–112). New York: New York University Press.

Zarit, S.H., & Whitlatch, C. (1992). Institutional placement: Phases of the transition. *The Gerontologist, 32,* 665–672.

RESOURCES

Generic versions of the following documents that we used in The Family Project are included in the Appendix:

- The initial introduction letter sent to participants

- The reminder letter sent to participants

- The information sheet handed out at the information sessions

- The evaluation instrument used for the pretest and posttest (Entrance/Exit Interview)

For any other requests for information about The Family Project, please contact

Terry Peak, M.S.W., Ph.D.
Director, Social Work Program
Department of Sociology, Social Work & Anthropology
Utah State University
0730 Old Main Hill
Logan, UT 84322
E-mail: tpeak@hass.usu.edu
Phone: 435-797-4080

5

Appendix

[Date]

Dear [name of facility] family member:

As you know, [name of facility] has a deep commitment to caring about our nursing home families. As part of that commitment, I am writing to inform you of an opportunity to become a participant in a project that [name of facility] will be cooperating with in conjunction with Dr. Terry Peak of the Social Work Program of Utah State University.

Dr. Peak has been awarded a 1-year grant from [research sponsor] to see if it is possible to improve the nursing home experience for family members of our residents. The project is called the Family Education and Support Program (The Family Project) and is an attempt to include the family more directly in the nursing home experience. The two goals of the project are

1. To see if providing a combination of helpful information and support group interaction to family members will help them enjoy their visits more

2. To improve the period of adjustment to the nursing home for both the residents and their families

Participation in The Family Project will entail group meetings with other [name of facility] family members once each week for 6 weeks. The meetings will each last about 1 hour and will include information about the aging process and how various diseases can affect normal aging, how a disease can affect your interaction with your relative, how to select activities during your visits that are appropriate to your relative's health condition, answers to specific questions you might have about [name of facility] procedures or staff, and opportunities to share your experiences and expertise with other family members.

A brief information meeting will be held in the Living Room at [name of facility] on [weekday date] at [time], and again on [weekend date] at [time], if you would like to learn more about this project. I am enclosing a business card for Dr. Peak if you would like to contact her directly with any questions you might have.

As always, if you have any questions about this project, or any other matter that affects [name of facility], please feel free to contact me.

Sincerely,
Facility Administrator

Enclosures

[Contact information here]

THE FAMILY EDUCATION AND
SUPPORT PROGRAM (THE FAMILY PROJECT)

We know that having a family member in a nursing home can be a stressful experience, so we are providing helpful information as well as the opportunity for social support with other family members just like you. Family members often complain that more could be done to make this difficult transition easier for them. In our meetings, we provide some of the assistance that family members ask for. We think this may result in you enjoying your nursing home visits more.

Family members can often benefit from specific education about what to expect from their relatives in terms of the relative's diagnosis. Sometimes, people need to be reminded that some distressing symptoms are *not* under the control of the resident. We also hope that family members will benefit from the social support provided by other family members in the group meetings. Families can feel isolated and as if they are the only ones who have to deal with these problems. The Family Project offers a safe place in which to discuss these issues with others who are experiencing the same problems.

The groups will meet once a week for approximately 1 hour at a time for 8 weeks. We will choose a time and a starting date that is most convenient for everyone.

The Family Project group sessions will include

1. Information about the aging process and how various diseases, especially dementia, can affect "normal" aging

2. Discussions about how families can most usefully interact with nursing home staff—what the visitor can expect from the staff and what the staff expects from visitors

3. Opportunities to share personal experiences and expertise with others in similar situations

4. Recommendations on how to communicate effectively with your relative

5. Suggestions for selecting a visit activity that is appropriate to your relative's condition and ideas for making the visit a positive experience for all involved

There are two experienced and trained social work students who will be helping. [Name 1] has worked at [name of facility] doing music therapy and is herself a caregiver. [Name 2] is also a family caregiver. Both have worked with the project for some time.

Because this is a research project funded by [research sponsor], family members who agree to participate in The Family Project will be asked to sign an informed consent form. In the form, we ask family members to agree to a brief entrance and exit interview. They are asked to keep track of the number and quality of their visits in a log that we supply and to rate their perception of the condition of their relative. We also ask permission to examine the nursing home charts in order to collect information about problem behaviors, use of medications, and use of restraints. We try to establish an individual goal with each participant at the pretest interview that will help us evaluate our success. Any information about either your family members or the relative in the nursing home will be kept strictly confidential. Project records will be code numbered and kept in a locked cabinet.

We hope that through The Family Project, family members can learn how to deal more effectively with their needs and the needs of their relative and to be able to better enjoy being a [name of facility] family member.

[Date]

Dear [name of facility] family member:

I am writing to remind you of your opportunity to participate in a support group research project being offered at [name of facility] in conjunction with [research sponsor]. We hope that through The Family Project, family members can learn how to deal more effectively with their own needs and the needs of their relative at [name of facility].

   Participation in The Family Project will mean group meetings with other [name of facility] family members once each week for 8 weeks. The meetings will each last about 1 hour and will provide answers to specific questions you might have about [name of facility] procedures or staff, information about the aging process and how various diseases can affect normal aging, information about how to select an activity during your visits that will be appropriate to your relative's health condition, and opportunities to share your experiences and expertise with other family members. One of our Family Project associates, [name of associate], will be contacting you to arrange for a brief preliminary interview so that we can provide you with information appropriate to your individual needs.

   Our first meeting will be in the Living Room at **[name of facility]** on **[date]** at **[time].** If you have any questions before that date, I am enclosing a business card so that you can contact me directly.

Sincerely,
Terry Peak, M.S.W., Ph.D.

Enclosures

Participant number: _____ Date: _____

ENTRANCE/EXIT INTERVIEW

The Relative in the Nursing Home

1. How long have you been involved with the care of your loved one?

2. What kinds of caregiving did you do for your loved one before nursing home admission?

3. What kinds of caregiving do you do for your loved one now that he/she is in [facility name]?

4. About how often do you visit your loved one at [facility name]?

5. Do you enjoy the visits?

   always   sometimes   rarely   never

6. How long has your loved one been at the nursing home?

7. What is your loved one's primary diagnosis?

8. What behaviors in your loved one (if any) are upsetting to you?

9. Would you like to be more involved in
the care of your loved one?

yes   no

If yes, in what ways?

10. How would you characterize how you feel about your loved
one now that he/she is in [facility name]?

worse than before   same as always   better than before

Social Support

11. How often (days per month) do you receive the following types
of social support from friends and relatives?

	Friends	Relatives
Telephone calls	_____	_____
Visits	_____	_____
Help	_____	_____
Other:	_____	_____

12. Are you satisfied with the help you receive from
Friends?

not at all   somewhat   a great deal

Relatives?

not at all   somewhat   a great deal

The Caregiver

13. How would you rate your health at present?

    excellent   good   fair   poor

14. Does your health get in the way of doing what you want to do?

    not at all   somewhat   a great deal

15. How much of the time during the past month did you feel downhearted and blue?

    all of the time   some of the time   none of the time

16. Is there some way the visitation process could be improved for you?

At Entrance

17. Can you think of any specific areas of information you would like us to provide to you during the support group?

18. What personal goal would you like to accomplish during the project?

19. Do you have any financial worries
    For yourself?   yes   no

    For your relative?   yes   no

20. Are you currently working?

    full time   part time   not working   retired   never worked

At Exit

21. Has there been any change in the behaviors
    in your relative that has been upsetting to you?

                                                           yes   no

    Explain:

22. Has there been any change in your attitude about
    being more involved in the care of your relative?

                                                           yes   no

    Explain:

23. How would you characterize how you feel about your relative
    today?

24. Do you feel that participating in the
    support group was beneficial?

                                                           yes   no

    Explain:

25. Did your feelings about being a caregiver change in any way?

26. Did this help with stress associated with caregiving?

27. During the group sessions, did you feel as if there was someone
    from whom you could get help?

Promoting Family Involvement in Long-Term Care Settings:
A Guide to Programs that Work, edited by Joseph E. Gaugler
© Copyright 2005 by Health Professions Press, Inc. All rights reserved.

28. Did the support group help you feel less alone?

29. Do you feel that you accomplished the
    personal goal you mentioned at your
    first interview [state goal]?

                                                        yes   no

    Explain:

6

Supporting Families of Persons with Dementia Living in Nursing Homes

The Family Visit Education Program

PHILIP MCCALLION

Families have long been recognized as critical contributors to the well-being of people with dementia (Cohen & Eisdorfer, 1986; Tune, Lucas-Blaustein, & Rovner, 1988). However, intervention strategies to improve the quality of life and help manage the problem behaviors of nursing home residents with dementia have been carried out almost exclusively by professional caregivers (Tirrito, 1997). Also, there has been a failure to recognize the impact of admission of a relative to a nursing home on the family caregivers themselves and its subsequent effect on the person with dementia (McCallion, Toseland, & Freeman, 1999). Although responsibility for physical care decreases after nursing home admission, family members often continue to experience a significant amount of stress (Naleppa, 1996). For example, family members often feel less supported. Moreover, admission can increase family members' feelings of guilt at not being able to meet the needs of the person with dementia. Also, emotional and tangible support from other family members and friends may decline after admission, thereby increasing the isolation of and sense of burden on the family member (McCallion, Toseland, & Freeman, 1999; Naleppa, 1996).

Family members are also reported to experience greater difficulties when they observe problem behaviors exhibited by the person with dementia following nursing home admission. Problem behaviors such as aggression and wandering are often more visible to family members after the person enters residential care (Stephens, Ogrocki, & Kinney, 1991). Indeed, as dementia progresses after placement, problem behaviors such as aggression and wandering often increase in frequency and intensity. Difficulties in coping with these behaviors and the potential embarrassment that can occur in front of staff and other families, coupled with the diminished capacity of the person with dementia to engage in conversation, make it difficult for many family members to conduct meaningful and satisfying interactions with residents. This often leads to frustration, reduced visitations, inappropriate interactions with the resident, and negative evaluations of nursing staff and the nursing home. Yet, there is also evidence that the pattern of interaction between family members and individuals with dementia may positively influence the extent and level of problem behaviors, and that assisting families to reduce critical and angry responses and to structure visits in a more supportive fashion has a positive impact on problem behaviors and encourages continued visiting (McCallion, Toseland, & Freeman, 1999).

Good intentions and efforts on the part of family members are often thwarted by poor understanding of the progression of dementia and by a lack of tools to respond more effectively. There is such an emphasis in communications by staff with family members on the declines associated with dementia that a sense of remaining strengths may be lost, and with it the value of continued efforts to support communication. This is one of the deficits that the Family Visit Education Program (FVEP) is designed to address. The intent was to develop an intervention that would be a tool both to reduce problem behaviors for the person with dementia and to support families sufficiently so that they would maintain, if not increase, their level of visiting.

DESCRIPTION OF THE INTERVENTION

The FVEP is a training program for families designed to address three areas:

1. Verbal and nonverbal communication

2. Use of memory aids

3. Responding to problem behaviors

FVEP is grounded in a stage-based understanding of the progression of dementia, primarily Alzheimer's disease, and in an understanding of how dementia affects both memory and communication skills. In offering tools for communication to family members, the FVEP seeks to emphasize the communication strengths that remain throughout the disease, encourage the family member to assume greater responsibility for the maintenance of interaction with the person as dementia progresses, and offer specific evidence-based tools to improve and support care (McCallion & Toseland, 1996; Toseland & McCallion, 1998).

The nursing home–based FVEP is generally delivered by a trainer over 8 weeks and includes four $1^1/2$-hour group sessions and three 1-hour family conferences. Group sessions are supplemented with individual family conferences to tailor intervention training to the level of dementia experienced by each resident. Family sessions have two components: a therapeutic observation of interaction between family members and the person with dementia with real-time feedback, and a face-to-face feedback session with individual family members not in the presence of the resident. The trainer usually observes the family member and resident interacting for 20–30 minutes and then provides an additional 15 minutes of feedback about his or her observations in a family meeting room (after the family member has completed his or her visit).

IMPLEMENTING THE INTERVENTION

Group Session 1

This session is designed to introduce the program. The rationale for FVEP is explained in detail. The impact of normal age-related changes on communication is also discussed, and information regarding the general and resident-specific progression of Alzheimer's disease or associated disorders is presented. Techniques to enhance communication with older people are described and demonstrated, such as ensuring that people who use eyeglasses and hearing aids are wearing them, reducing background noise and other distractions, and ensuring that there is adequate lighting.

Family members have an opportunity to share their experiences, frustrations, and suggestions with each other and with the FVEP leader. Strains they experience when visiting their relative with dementia are discussed, along with the belief that improved interaction strategies may have a positive impact on the resident. The resident's stage of dementia also is discussed. The negative impact that dementia has had on the resident's memory and communication skills, and the communication strengths that remain in the resident, are also discussed. In addition, visiting family members are given the opportunity to assess and discuss their own communication styles, strengths, and needs.

Group Session 2

In the second group session, family members receive assistance in techniques for communicating more effectively, verbally and nonverbally, with people experiencing mild, moderate, and severe dementia. A portion of the session is spent discussing why techniques such as correcting, reorienting, ignoring, and attempting to engage in a rational conversation often do not work, and why they may actually increase agitation. Emphasis is placed on opening lines of communication by viewing the behavior of the person with dementia as an attempt to communicate, recognizing the dementia-related communication deficits that are experienced, and making maximum use of remaining communication strengths.

Family members also role-play and practice five nonverbal and ten verbal techniques found to be helpful in fostering supportive interactions with individuals with dementia. The techniques are drawn from Feil (2003), Hoffman and Platt (1991), Rau (1993), and Weiner (1991). A strong emphasis is placed on recognizing and responding to nonverbal responses received from the person with dementia that family members might otherwise miss. Nonverbal techniques include

1. *Relaxing.* Family members are taught to release their own emotions before interacting with the resident by using a deep-breathing relaxation technique. This helps family members avoid becoming anxious, frustrated, or annoyed while listening to and interacting with the resident who, because of dementia, seems to make no sense or behaves in an irrational fashion.

2. *Maintaining eye contact.*

3. *Using a clear, low, loving tone of voice.*

4. *Touching.* Family members are taught that because people with dementia often have diminished visual and auditory acuity, they

often appreciate feeling the touch of another human being. Family members may need to reevaluate the resident's comfort level with touching.

5. *Mirroring.* Family members are taught to match the resident's motions and emotions to convey understanding and acceptance of the resident's feelings and attempts to communicate.

Certain verbal techniques also help to foster communication with people with dementia. Instead of conveying frustration, disapproval, or a desire to "calm" the person, the verbal techniques emphasize responding with empathy. During the group and individual sessions, guidance is offered to family members on the selection of verbal techniques that are most appropriate for each stage of dementia. The verbal techniques are as follows:

1. *Being supportive and nonconfrontational.* Family members are encouraged to use nonthreatening words to build trust and to avoid being critical of the resident. For example, "I know you are upset; let me clean up this mess."

2. *Asking simple, concrete questions.* Family members are taught to break down what they say into simple, concrete questions to promote communication. For example, "I know you are upset; is there too much noise here?"

3. *Increasing time for responses.* Family members are taught to talk slowly, to pause frequently, and to repeat key phrases when conversing with the resident because the reaction times of a person with dementia are often greatly slowed. For example, "Maybe there is too much noise here. . . . Too much noise?"

4. *Structuring, focusing, and simplifying conversation.* Family members are taught to take more responsibility for structuring and focusing conversations to facilitate the resident's use of remaining cognitive and communication skills, and to simplify instructions about tasks to remove demands that are beyond the ability of the resident. For example, "I think it is a little noisy here. What do you think? Noisy, isn't it? Do you think I should turn down the TV? I'll turn down the TV, OK?"

5. *Encouraging and guiding.* Family members are taught how to use verbal and nonverbal cues to encourage and stimulate the resident

to continue to communicate and ways to guide the resident through communication sequences and activities that he or she is having trouble completing. They are also taught techniques that help the resident to continue to do things for him- or herself. For example, "Why don't I hold the sweater to make it easier for you to put it on."

6. *Rephrasing and paraphrasing.* Family members are taught to repeat the resident's basic message using the same key words, tone of voice, and cadence of speech. This encourages continued communication by enabling the resident to hear what he or she said, by giving the person time to gather his or her thoughts in preparation for continuing the conversation, and by ensuring that the message being conveyed is understood as intended. For example, "Have I got this right? You're saying you want to go outside?"

7. *Reminiscing.* Family members are taught to encourage the resident to explore and express pleasant memories from the past. Family members are also taught not to focus on the accuracy of these memories but instead to encourage the resident to express him- or herself. For example, "So tell me about when we went to Miami" (the trip was actually with someone else).

8. *Avoiding ambiguity.* Family members are taught to accept words that have no meaning to others and to respond by using ambiguous or vague terms in their responses to such words so that communication with the resident can be maintained. For example, in response to "The dim shouted at me," the family member might respond, "He did! What happened next?"

9. *Identifying the preferred sense.* Family members are taught to identify the resident's preferred sense and to communicate in terms of that sense (Feil, 2003). For example, if the resident repeatedly communicates by using visual images such as "I see it over there. It makes me nervous," family members might be encouraged to respond with a simple question such as "What else do you see? What color is it?" which encourages the resident to use the preferred sense: sight.

10. *Linking the behavior with the unmet human need.* Individuals with dementia express basic needs through their behaviors; family members are taught to identify and respond to these needs.

The remainder of the meeting is spent practicing these techniques through role plays. In consultation with the FVEP leader, each family member or family group identifies and practices specific alternative verbal and nonverbal interaction techniques they wish to try with their relative with dementia. The leader emphasizes selecting techniques that are appropriate for the stage of dementia and building upon each resident's remaining communication strengths (see Table 6.1).

Individual Conference 1

The FVEP leader spends 30–60 minutes with each family member or family group. During the first half of the visit, the FVEP leader observes interactions of family members with the resident with dementia. Later, the leader discusses his or her observations, praising efforts to maintain communication and assisting family members to identify specific concerns and problems that they would like to address through the program. In particular, the FVEP leader helps family members identify barriers that prevent them from communicating more effectively and how to overcome these barriers. For example, a family member might identify that, when she visits after the facility's dinner hour, the resident always complains that she was not given any dinner to eat (although it has been verified that she did eat the meal). During the course of the visit, the resident then becomes very agitated and the family member finds the experience very upsetting. During the first half of the individual conference, the FVEP leader might observe the family member's attempts to reorient the resident and the agitation and frustrations that result. The FVEP leader and the family member might then agree to work on this communication barrier.

During the second half of the individual conference, the FVEP leader then assists the family member to identify and understand verbal and nonverbal messages conveyed by the resident and to implement the alternative verbal and nonverbal interaction strategies he or she has chosen and practiced in group session 2. The family member, for example, might select being supportive and nonconfrontational as the approach she would like to try with the resident who complains about not having received dinner and to try distracting the resident by incorporating reminiscence about favorite dinners and the importance of dinnertime. The FVEP leader might then observe the family member implementing the chosen communication strategy, give feedback,

Table 6.1. Key communication strategies for each stage of dementia

Communicating with Persons with Early Stage Dementia
  Use simple, direct language.
  Let them teach you their attention span.
  Use different words and provide more information.
  Avoid talking for and filling in words.
  Allow time for processing.
  Introduce a topic, summarize what you want to say, and then give details.
  Reminisce—talk about things in each person's past.
  Allow them to express their feelings.
  Express your support and caring.
  Repeat important messages.
  Use memory aids.
  Give specific instructions and information before it is needed.

Communicating with Persons with Middle Stage Dementia
  Speak to them only when you are visible.
  Use their name, and give your name.
  Avoid saying, "Do you know who I am?"
  Use overemphasis, gestures, facial expressions and pointing to familiar objects to support
    what you're saying.
  Make sure you have been understood.
  Wait for them to respond.
  If they do not respond—repeat once.
  If not understood, use a different, simpler way to express something rather than repeating
    over and over.
  Use people's names, not "he" or "she."
  Offer a predictable routine.
  Offer familiar activities.
  Put labels/signs on things that are important to their daily life.
  Don't take their behavior personally.
  Listen and repeat what was said to be sure you have understood.
  Encourage and praise them.
  Use all available cues to understand what they are trying to communicate.
  Avoid sudden changes in topic.
  Avoid long and complex sentences.

Communicating with Persons with Severe/Late Stage Dementia
  Speak to them only when you are visible.
  Begin by using their name.
  Give your own name.
  Smile.
  Keep your voice low, affectionate, and subdued.
  Use overemphasis, gestures, and facial expressions to convey your message.
  Speak very slowly and very clearly.
  Assume the person hears you.
  Do not speak to others as if the person with dementia is not in the room.
  Keep talking even if there is no response.
  Use touch.
  Respond to seemingly meaningless speech.
  Look for nonverbal messages.
  Listen to music, read aloud.
  Always say goodbye.

From McCallion, P. (2004). *Facing the challenges of dementia* [CD-ROM]. Albany, NY: New York State Office of Children & Family Services; reprinted by permission.

discuss successes and frustrations, and offer further advice and encouragement.

Group Session 3

In the third group session, family members are introduced to memory aids. This includes working with nursing home staff on labeling the resident's possessions with the name of the possession; putting written and graphic signs on important locations in the unit, such as the bathroom and the dining room; and developing a *personal memory chart or album.* Personal memory albums are small photo albums with easily turned pages with a photograph of a key memory on one page and a short statement about that memory on the facing page. On personal memory charts, the same types of photographs and statements are placed on large, laminated pieces of cardboard posted on the resident's bedroom walls at heights that take into account whether the resident is ambulatory or spends most of the day in a wheelchair. Personal memory albums and charts are designed to promote positive interactions and to focus on maintaining previously learned information rather than imparting new information. The memory items address facts that are important to the resident, information on conversation topics the resident likes or wants to talk about, and facts that the resident often gets confused. Family members are taught to use personal memory albums and charts consistently and frequently.

To address facts that are important to the resident with dementia, information on some of the following topics might be included in a personal memory album or chart:

1. *The person:* name, age, place of birth, schools attended, occupation

2. *The person's family:* names of family members and their relationship to the resident

3. *The person's daily life:* days and times for important events

4. *People with whom the person now lives:* the names of roommates, neighbors down the hall, and other residents who attend the same activities

5. *People who work at the nursing home:* names of certified nursing assistants (CNAs), nurses, social workers, activity directors, and other staff whom the resident sees regularly on the unit

With respect to conversation topics, family members identify three topics that the resident likes or wants to talk about. These topics may be from the resident's current life or from his or her past. Topics that relate to the resident's family, past activities, and past interests, as well as topics that the resident him- or herself continues to attempt to discuss, are often used. Family members are encouraged to talk to staff and to other family members to identify conversation topics. Finally, the resident's forgetfulness of key facts often makes communication difficult. To limit the impact of forgetfulness and confusion, key daily and weekly events such as meals, appointments, and family visits are often included in the personal memory album or chart.

Family members practice developing a personal memory album or chart during the third session. The FVEP leader reviews and has the family members role-play use of the personal memory album or chart in accordance with the following guidelines:

1. The family member should point to the appropriate section of the personal memory album or chart when discussing the person, event, or topic to which it relates, even when the resident appears to understand the family member's words.

2. The family member should encourage the resident to point to the appropriate section of the personal memory album or chart when discussing the person, event, or topic to which it relates.

3. The personal memory album or chart should be used as often as possible in interactions with the resident.

To support continued communication by residents with dementia who also have visual impairments, the development of a personal memory audiotape is also demonstrated as part of this session. As recommended by Woods and Ashley (1995), key family members and friends are asked to "converse" on an audiotape with the resident about cherished memories, loved ones, family anecdotes, and other favored experiences from the resident's life. It is likely that these are events and people that the resident will enjoy talking about. The tape has soundless intervals during which the resident and family members discuss what was shared. Contributors to the tape are also often asked to include a segment on key events in the resident's day-to-day life and facts that the resident tends to forget.

In advance of the second individual conference, family members are instructed to gather materials for a personal memory album or chart.

Individual Conference 2

The FVEP leader again spends time with each participating family member. The leader reviews the personal memory album or chart materials. A preliminary album or chart is developed, and the leader observes the family member introducing it to the resident with dementia. In the example of the resident who complains of not receiving her dinner, the family member might decide to include in the person's personal memory chart the statement "I ate dinner today at 6:00 P.M." and a picture of the person sitting in the dining room eating dinner. In addition, the family member might continue to use the verbal technique of being supportive and nonconfrontational by pointing to another picture on the chart, which encourages the resident to talk about this cherished memory. The leader might then give the family member feedback on the use of the personal memory chart to convey this information, discuss successes and frustrations in implementing the technique, and offer further advice and encouragement on developing and modifying the memory aid.

Group Session 4

In response to family members' requests for specific strategies to address problem behaviors, during the fourth session the FVEP leader outlines a three-step communications-based approach to problem behaviors:

1. Find and respond to the need.

2. Find the memory.

3. Ensure safety.

Find and Respond to the Need

Family members are trained to look for four possible sources of need-related problem behaviors:

1. Agitated or problem behaviors often occur when an important basic need is not being met. For example,

    • Is the person hungry or thirsty?

    • Does the person need to be moved in the wheelchair or bed?

    • Is the person soiled?

- Is the person angry, depressed, sad, or exhausted?

- Is the person ill?

- Is the person frustrated by a task or from not being able to communicate?

2. Something in the room or nursing home may be causing the behavior. For example,

- Is the room too hot or too cold?

- Is the room too bright or too dark?

- Is there too much noise in or outside of the room?

3. Staff, family members, or someone else is doing something that bothers the person with dementia. For example,

- Is someone near the person acting angry, irritated, or bored?

- Has someone rearranged the person's favored possessions?

- Does the person want to be left alone for a while?

4. The behavior is not the problem. For example,

- Is the person wandering because he or she likes to exercise?

- Is the person agitated because he or she is bored?

- Is a task that is being asked of the person too difficult and frustrating?

Strategies role-played by family members to discover the nature of the need include 1) asking yes/no questions to narrow down what is agitating the resident, 2) interpreting the resident's gestures and other nonverbal signs, 3) trying to look at the situation through the resident's eyes, and 4) recalling what caused similar incidents in the past.

Find the Memory

The leader explains that some experts believe that as people with dementia connect more and more with their past, they also revisit past conflicts and problems, and that this can cause agitation (Feil, 2003). Strategies that are role-played with family members include listening for familiar names and events and asking simple questions that encourage and assist the resident to explain what is upsetting him or her.

Ensure Safety

The FVEP leader explains and role-plays with family members techniques designed to maintain safety for both the resident and the staff:

- Staying calm because this will be calming for the resident

- Speaking in soothing tones and keeping all body language non-threatening

- Distracting the resident with a favorite activity

- Getting help if there is a danger of injury to the family member or to the resident

Individual Conference 3

The FVEP leader again assists each family member at a time when problem behaviors are likely to occur with the resident with dementia, such as during mealtimes or dressing/bathing. Responding with some of the recommended strategies may continue to prove difficult for family members to implement. The final session provides an opportunity to practice any techniques family members are not yet comfortable with and to reconsider what techniques might be most helpful for the resident. In the example of the resident who complains that she has not received dinner, during the discussion of problem behaviors during the fourth group session, the family member might point out that she and staff members have observed how heartily the person usually eats at dinner (i.e., "she cleans the plate"). The FVEP leader might ask if there is a possibility that the resident is still hungry. The family member might indicate that she does not know and acknowledge that she has never attempted to find out. The family member may decide that the response to a problem behavior she wishes to try during the third individual conference is "find the need." Using questions that will result in yes/no answers, the family member might gently ask if the resident is still hungry. If the resident indicates she is, then the family member might plan to work with nursing and dietary staff to address this problem. The family member might continue to be supportive and nonconfrontational through the use of the personal memory chart to assist the resident to recall that she did have dinner. The FVEP leader might observe the family member implementing the communication and memory aid approaches she has learned in each of the sessions, provide the family member with feedback, discuss successes and frustrations in implementing the techniques, and offer further advice and encouragement.

KEY IMPLEMENTATION CONCERNS

Key implementation concerns revolve around the quality of the materials used and the quality of the leader delivering the intervention. A manualized version of the intervention is available that consists of a leader manual, a family participant workbook that includes reviews of materials shared and assignments, and a "train-the-trainer" videotape covering key components of FVEP training and delivery (see Resources at the end of the chapter).

In its initial offering, FVEP was delivered by a master's-level practitioner experienced in working with residents with dementia and their families. This is also recommended for any future leaders. Each leader participated in four half-day training sessions that included 1) education on the stages of dementia and on available resources, designed to equip the leaders to respond knowledgeably to questions raised by families; 2) a review of the verbal and nonverbal communication strategies that are effective with individuals with moderate to severe dementia; 3) role-playing and practice of these strategies; 4) instruction on developing and utilizing memory aids; and 5) approaches to training families, including agendas for individual and group instructional sessions, the design and use of slides/overheads in group sessions, and techniques for conducting observations and providing constructive feedback. The four half days of training relied on the leader manual, participant workbook, and training videotape. Also, prior to beginning the training, the practitioner was required to do some background reading (Feil, 2003; Hoffman & Platt, 1991; Rau, 1993; Weiner, 1991). It will be possible for future leaders to sufficiently orient themselves to the intervention using the manuals and videotape that are available.

EVALUATION

A systematic evaluation of the FVEP training program has been conducted (McCallion, Toseland, & Freeman, 1999). In a randomized, controlled trial, 66 residents with dementia and their primary visiting family members were drawn from five skilled nursing homes and assigned to treatment and control conditions. Residents were assessed for 1) psychosocial functioning, 2) depression, 3) agitated behavior, and 4) degree of positive social interaction. Nursing staff members were assessed for changes in the time and methods used to manage problem behaviors. Visiting family members were assessed for 1) dementia management skills, 2) extent of perceived caregiving hassles, and 3) satisfaction with visits. It was found that FVEP was effective in reducing residents' problem behaviors and in decreasing their symptoms of depression and irritability. FVEP was also effective in improving the way family members and other visitors communicated with residents, but, with the exception of reducing the use of mechanical restraints, it was not effective in changing nurses' management of residents' behavior problems (McCallion, Toseland, & Freeman, 1999).

A version of the FVEP program was also developed for use with CNAs (McCallion, Toseland, Lacey, & Banks, 1999). In evaluating this program, it was not possible to randomize individual subjects. Instead, four units of residents and associated staff in two nursing homes were randomly assigned to conditions. In total, 88 CNAs and 105 residents with dementia were involved in the study. Again, there were significant improvements in measures of resident well-being, and staff reported significant increases in knowledge of effective communication-based caregiving responses. A significant decrease in staff turnover also occurred. A partial crossover design was used in the CNA study, permitting the intervention to be offered to the control units after a period of time. Data were again collected, and the findings for the original treatment group were replicated when the control group received the intervention. The findings here reinforce the value of the materials shared in FVEP.

The resident measures used in the two studies appeared to be particularly sensitive in detecting changes over time for a population in which positive changes are often difficult to discern. It appears that the following instruments may be worth considering by practitioners interested in assessing the impact of their interventions for persons with dementia:

Cornell Scale for Depression in Dementia (CSDD): The CSDD is a 19-item instrument that assesses signs and symptoms of depression in the following areas: 1) mood-related signs, 2) behavioral disturbance, 3) physical signs, 4) cyclic functions, and 5) ideational disturbance. The CSDD is clinician-administered and uses information obtained from both the resident and the nursing home staff. The scale has good interrater reliability (alpha = .67) and internal consistency (alpha = .84), as well as good sensitivity (Alexopoulos, Abrams, Young, & Shamoian, 1988).

Cohen-Mansfield Agitation Inventory (CMAI): The CMAI is a 30-item instrument that is utilized to measure agitated behavior of elders. The 30 items encompass three broad categories of behavior: 1) aggressive behavior, 2) physically nonaggressive behavior, and 3) verbally agitated behavior (Cohen-Mansfield, Marx, & Rosenthal, 1989). The occurrence of behaviors during a previous 2-week period were rated by nurse managers on each shift on 7-point scales ranging from never (1) to several times an hour (7). The CMAI has good interrater reliability (alpha = .88) and validity.

Multidimensional Observation Scale for Elderly Subjects (MOSES): Three subscales from the 24-item short form of the MOSES—Disorientation, Irritability, and Withdrawal—appeared particularly useful. Internal consistency reliabilities for the subscales averaged .80, interrater reliabilities ranged from a low of .72 to a high of .97, and the concurrent validity of the subscales was established (Helmes, Csapo, & Short, 1987; Pruchno, Kleban, & Resch, 1988).

All of these instruments appear to be sensitive to change over time and have demonstrated considerable utility in the periodic reassessment and monitoring of individuals with dementia who should be benefiting from FVEP.

IMPLICATIONS AND CONCLUSIONS

It is frequently challenging in dementia care to find evidence-based psychosocial interventions, and those interventions that are available tend to be targeted exclusively to the person with dementia. Yet, family members continue to have a significant impact on the quality of life for individuals with dementia and may continue to carry their own distress from the experience of dementia in the relative following nursing home admission. FVEP offers an advantage in that there is systematically gathered evidence to support its use. Its manuals and its approach to training may also contain lessons for training in other aspects of dementia care. At the very least, FVEP models both how materials are developed and how training is delivered in order to exert the maximum impact on improving care for people with dementia living in nursing homes.

REFERENCES

Alexopoulos, G., Abrams, R., Young, R., & Shamoian, C. (1988). Cornell Scale for Depression in Dementia. *Journal of Biological Psychology, 23,* 271–284.

Cohen, S., & Eisdorfer, C. (1986). *The loss of self: A family resource for the care of Alzheimer's disease and related disorders.* New York: Norton.

Cohen-Mansfield, J., Marx, M., & Rosenthal, A. (1989). A description of agitation in a nursing home. *Journals of Gerontology. Series A, Biological Sciences and Medical Sciences, 44,* M77–M84.

Feil, N. (2003). *The validation breakthrough* (2nd ed.). Baltimore: Health Professions Press.

Helmes, E., Csapo, K., & Short, J. (1987). Standardization and validation of the Multidimensional Observation Scale for Elderly Subjects (MOSES). *Journal of Gerontology, 42,* 395–405.

Hoffman, S., & Platt, C. (1991). *Comforting the confused: Strategies for managing dementia.* New York: Springer.

McCallion, P. (2004). *Facing the challenges of dementia* [CD-Rom]. Albany, NY: New York State Office of Children & Family Services.

McCallion, P., & Toseland, R.W. (1996). *Family Visit Education Program.* Unpublished leader manual, participant workbook, and training videotape, School of Social Welfare, University at Albany, NY.

McCallion, P., Toseland, R.W., & Freeman, K. (1999). An evaluation of a family visit education program. *Journal of the American Geriatrics Society, 47,* 203–214.

McCallion, P., Toseland, R.W., Lacey, D., & Banks, S. (1999). Educating nursing assistants to communicate more effectively with nursing home residents with dementia. *The Gerontologist, 39,* 546–558.

Naleppa, M.J. (1996). Families and the institutionalized elderly: A review. *Journal of Gerontological Social Work, 27,* 73–86.

Pruchno, R., Kleban, H., & Resch, N. (1988). Psychometric assessment of the Multidimensional Observation Scale for Elderly Subjects (MOSES). *Journal of Gerontology, 43,* 164–169.

Rau, M. (1993). *Coping with communication challenges in Alzheimer's disease.* San Diego: Singular.

Stephens, M., Ogrocki, P., & Kinney, J. (1991). Sources of stress for family caregivers of institutionalized dementia patients. *Journal of Applied Gerontology, 10,* 328–342.

Tirrito, T. (1997). Mental health problems and behavioral disruptions in nursing homes: Are social workers prepared to provide needed services? *Journal of Gerontological Social Work, 27,* 73–86.

Toseland, R., & McCallion, P. (1998). *Maintaining communication with persons with dementia.* New York: Springer.

Tune, L., Lucas-Blaustein, M., & Rovner, B. (1988). Psychosocial interventions. In L. Jarvik & C. Hutner-Winograd (Eds.), *Treatments for the Alzheimer patient: The long haul* (pp. 123–136). New York: Springer.

Weiner, M. (1991). *The dementias: Diagnosis and management.* Washington, DC: American Psychiatric Press.

Woods, P., & Ashley, J. (1995). Simulated presence therapy: Using selected memories to manage problem behaviors in Alzheimer's disease patients. *Geriatric Nursing, 16,* 9–14.

RESOURCE

For information and more details about FVEP training manuals and materials, as well as issues related to the implementation and evaluation of FVEP, please contact

Philip McCallion, Ph.D.
Center for Excellence in Aging Services
University at Albany
135 Western Avenue
Albany, NY 12222
E-mail: mcclion@albany.edu
Telephone: 518-442-5347
Fax: 518-442-3830

III

Family-Staff Partnerships

7

The Family Stories Workshop

KENNETH HEPBURN AND WAYNE A. CARON

This chapter describes the Family Stories Workshop, a project the authors of this chapter undertook to use narrative, or story, as a way to bridge the multiple gaps that can open between family members and residential care staff when a person with dementia moves from a situation of family caregiving to one of residential care. The chapter deals mainly with the "how to" of the program, describing the structure and techniques the authors employed to prepare family members to tell to staff the stories of relatives who could no longer recall, let alone frame and narrate, their own life histories.

The Family Stories Workshop drew its relevance from two main sources. First, people with dementia are the principal clients of residential care facilities and are likely to constitute an even greater proportion of the residential population in the future, in part because the prevalence of dementing disorders continues to increase. At present, at least 4.5 million Americans are affected by these disorders, and, by some estimates, this number will grow to nearly 14 million by 2050 (Alzheimer's Association, 2004). Prevalence estimates of dementia in nursing homes range from 25% to 75% (Magaziner et al., 2000). Although the norm for dementia care is family and home care, this care generally is provided only up to a certain point in the progress of the disease. At some point, daily care tasks exceed the capacity of the family caregiver, and more formal help is sought, help that includes a housing component as well as more extensive hands-on care. Whether it is a husband or a wife who is living with a spouse with dementia or an adult child who looks in on a parent with dementia on a regular basis, a moment may arrive when the caregiver acknowledges that admission to residential care has to occur.

The situation of admission—whether to an assisted living facility or a nursing home—constitutes the second main source of relevance for the Family Stories Workshop. The moment of admission for a person with a dementing illness brings with it the intersection of concerns of three sets of actors: families, care staff members, and the newly admitted person.

Admission of a relative with dementia by family members is usually not without conflict. For family caregivers, the act of admitting a spouse or parent (or other relation) to a residential care facility often involves a complex set of emotions. It is well understood that the physical and emotional investment in caregiving exacts a massive toll on caregivers (e.g., Pinquart & Sorensen, 2003a, 2003b; Vitaliano, Zhang, & Scanlan, 2003), so the admission comes at a time of fatigue and depletion. Anecdotes abound regarding the promises people make to relatives never to admit them to residential care, so the potential for guilt is considerable. More to the point, from the perspective of the Family Stories Workshop, families are typically heavily invested both in the quality of life of a relative with disability and in the strategies they have employed to secure a positive life experience for the relative when he or she still lived in the community. Families, therefore, are frequently protective of their relatives in new residences and are dubious—if not downright suspicious—about the people who take over providing the care that they used to provide. Moreover, placement does not appear to lift the load from family caregivers; burden and distress levels remain high in caregivers even after admission (e.g., Aneshensel, Pearlin, Mullan, Zarit, & Whitlatch, 1995; Schulz et al., 2004; Tornatore & Grant, 2002). One possible explanation for the continued sense of burden that might contribute to the tension that families feel with residential staff is role loss for families. For so long, family members played a central role in the resident's well-being. Now what is their role? How can they continue to contribute to the resident's well-being?

The addition of a new resident in a care facility changes, by necessity, the ecology of the facility. Staff members—whose overriding role it is to maintain the capacity of the facility to maximize the quality of life of its residents—must undertake a set of assessments and adjustments to accommodate and care for a person with little or no capacity for self-report. Although care staff and people with dementia can form bonds of fondness and delight, they cannot form bonds rooted in an appreciation by staff of the historical context of the person. Unless provided in some other way, the personal history, or the story, of the individual does not enter into the equation of bonding between staff and residents with dementia. Given the apparent satisfaction and closeness that staff members gain from knowing the persons for whom they care (e.g., Heiselman & Noelker, 1991; Sumaya-Smith, 1995), this gap in knowledge can detract from the rewards staff derive from their work. Residents—particularly residents with dementia—often come with families attached, and the process of arriving at terms of agreement with families is a significant and stressful part of the work staff members may face (e.g., see Rubin & Shuttlesworth, 1983; Schwarz & Vogel, 1990; Shuttlesworth, Rubin, & Duffy, 1982).

Finally, admission to residential care most of all affects the person with dementia. Although the art of the residential care of individuals with dementia has clearly developed over time, the move to a new residence presents a serious challenge to people with an already severely compromised capacity to respond to environmental demands. However poorly perceived and understood they might have been, the routines of the person's community environment had been honed over time and must have provided some form of comfort and security. Family caregivers had evolved strategies to deal with those times when their relative with cognitive impairment was overtaxed; they had learned the treats and tricks that produced moments of calm or delight, and they could spot the nuanced gesture that signaled a need to slow down or back off. Now, in a strange new place, a group of strangers—skilled, but strangers nonetheless—have to quickly develop a repertoire for caring that fits this individual and allows him or her to have a day-to-day life that is as pleasant and nonthreatening as possible.

THE FAMILY STORIES WORKSHOP INTERVENTION

When the chapter authors developed the Family Stories Workshop, they envisioned it as targeted to the early moments of admission, a time that has the potential to be unsatisfying and unfulfilling for all concerned. They did not see it as a panacea, but thought it could contribute both to fostering meaningful communication and to providing one basis for forming relationships between families and staff that would be beneficial both for them and for the new resident (Hepburn et al., 1997).

The Family Stories Workshop is a structured approach to the development of brief stories. The stories are intended to represent, in vignette form, important elements of the essence of the person who can no longer represent his or her own self. Over time, the chapter authors came to understand that representation can take forms other than stories; objects and rituals, for example, can provide insight into the person. The basic intent of developing these representations was that, at some point early in the new residency of the person, the family would meet with care staff and convey this representation—speak for the person to tell the staff who the person was and is.

THE FAMILY STORIES WORKSHOP PROCESS

The Family Stories Workshop process was focused on a specific end point: the recounting of a resident's story by a family member to the nursing home staff members who provide the care for that resident. This event itself has meaning and importance for a number of reasons. First, the nature of performance focuses attention on the performer. Placing the family member at the center of the performance highlights the family member as an authority about the resident—and therefore as a potential resource in the care of the resident. Second, the performance can be viewed as a rite of passage, a moment embodying the transition of care from that provided primarily by families to that provided in a formal and institutional setting. Again, the family member takes the lead role in this passing of care; he or she is the one who delivers the story of the person into the care of the listening staff. Finally, the performance is a way of modeling communication between family and staff. The dialogue that hopefully ensues following the formal presentation of the story could be conducted as a conversation between equals, a conversation in which the authority and expertise of the family member would be acknowledged as having value and status equivalent to that of the professional and paraprofessional care staff.

The Family Stories Workshop process was conducted within a group coaching model. A professional facilitator led each of the workshops. Members of the nursing home staff (variously, nurse educators, social workers, and a chaplain) regularly joined the leaders from the academic side (a gerontologist and a family counselor) during the field test of the program. Whereas the role of the facilitators was to maintain the agenda of the process itself (described later in the chapter) in order to foster a high level of participation and interaction, to assure that all workshop members were sticking to the process, and to participate actively in the process, the role of the family members in the workshop was key to the overall success of the workshops. Perhaps because group members shared a sense of something like anticipatory stage fright, camaraderie developed very quickly among them. Because the workshop process involved a gradual uncovering and unfolding of facts and feelings about the resident's life, the sense of appreciation that the group provided, even for mundane details about the resident, was of great value in prompting participants to continue the work of assembling information and shaping it into stories. Thus, group participation and encouragement helped to establish and reinforce the creative momentum of participants. As material emerged about the residents whose stories were being constructed, the group exercised a key editorial function. The group's reaction to materials—either direct verbal reaction or, perhaps more evocative, subtle nonverbal reaction—often cued family members about whether to continue to use the materials. Finally, the group played an invaluable role in providing positive reinforcement to members as the stories became more and more crystallized and refined.

The Family Stories Workshop followed a sequenced process. The process itself was grounded in two basic assumptions. The first of these is that a story is more than a list of facts. That is, the aim of the process—a narrative—was to express something of the essence of the person, and, although events and occurrences might form the backdrop of the person's life, the meaning of the person is not adequately or accurately expressed by only those facts. The second assumption was that although most people can tell stories—with more or less natural grace and an innate sense of theater—the facilitators were far less certain that most people naturally know how to construct stories or to craft them into an engaging performance. Thus, they established a process designed to accomplish, in sequence, a number of ends:

- Identify story materials and sources for story materials.

- Develop in participants a sense of what a life story is about, what it typically entails, and how to craft it.

- Select key story materials.

- Facilitate the crafting of stories.

- Permit rehearsal and editing of the stories.

- Organize the performance of the stories.

In the following sections, the aims and techniques of the various elements of the sequenced process are presented in terms of three main components: fact gathering, story crafting, and performance shaping.

Fact Gathering

Because biography, which was essentially what the stories were, is grounded in the facts and particulars of a person's life, the Family Stories Workshop began its story development process with exercises designed to accumulate and assemble facts about the life of the resident whose story was to be told. Two main exercises comprised the fact-gathering phase of the workshop: genograms and time lines. Both were designed to yield material that had received little or no authorial influence.

The genogram exercise was conducted during the initial session of the workshop. Participants were given no advance notice that this exercise would be done, and so there was no expectation that participants would have prepared for it. The purpose of the genogram exercise was to provide a historical and familial context for the life of the resident. Typically, participants were asked to place their relative in the context of two prior generations (i.e., going back to grandparents). The form of the genogram sought information about members of the resident's family through the generations; thus, there was interest not only in maternal and paternal grandparents but in siblings as well. The same information was sought for parents. The basic idea was to prompt the family member to recall the background of the resident and to invoke the kind, size, setting, and adventures of the generations that produced the resident. Moving forward, the genogram sought information about the resident's own family life. Thus, the exercise elicited information about marital history (including family history on the spouse's side) and about the generations that flowed from that history.

As anyone who has ever worked with genograms knows, what emerges from these seemingly mechanical exercises is typically highly evocative. Migrations, tragedies, and undying conflicts are present in almost every family, and experiences often have very potent influences on the lives of family members. In many cases in our field study, for example, immigration played a big part in the lives of those whose stories were to be told. In some cases, the residents themselves immigrated; in other cases it was their parents. Likewise, the history of relationships within families was often marked by early death or divorces and remarriages, leading to complicated intergenerational relationships. In all of these cases, culture or family served as the backdrop against which many lives were lived. For example, one of the residents was raised by parents who moved as adults to a Swedish-speaking community in the United States; her life, until the time she left her small town and came to an urban area, was fully conducted in Swedish among Swedish speakers. Although she learned English in school, it was not her real first language; and although she was born and raised in America, it could accurately be said that it was not her native country. Thus, from the genogram exercise alone, the family member and the whole group became aware that, whatever would unfold in this story, it would have to have as a key theme the idea of a stranger in a strange land, a Ruth among the alien corn. Similarly, the mere representation of a resident in terms of a genogram that portrayed his two marriages and two sets of children alerted the family member and the group that the management of conflict and relationships would likely be an important component of the story that would develop.

The genogram exercise not only served to introduce the workshop participants to the generational facts about the residents, but also served as a safe icebreaker for the group and, in many instances, provided workshop participants with connections to each other (e.g., through shared ethnic backgrounds). Beyond this, the genogram alerted participants to what they did not know about their relatives (e.g., children who told the story of their parents often had only cursory knowledge of their great-grandparent's generation). It helped them to identify where their research ought to focus to have a better picture of these facts. In addition, by portraying the members of the family, the exercise helped participants identify resources within the family who might prove helpful in filling out the picture. Many adult children reported visits and phone calls to aunts and uncles seeking more information, details, and insight into the life and character of the relative whose story was to be told. As a matter of group process, as participants garnered more information about family history, they were always welcome to bring that to the group and add to the group's picture of the resident.

The Family Stories Workshop used a decade-by-decade time line as the second fact-gathering exercise. In this exercise, participants divided the resident's life into decades (ages birth–10, 11–20, and so forth) up to the present and filled in the key facts of the resident's life during each decade. To complete this exercise, participants were free to use whatever sources they could find: diaries, family lore, records, key informants within (and beyond) the family, and their own memory. In many instances, the material for the first two decades was not very complete, and it was often not very dramatic; people were born, went to school, and, in some cases, left home. In other cases, highly significant events (e.g., the sudden death of a parent, a major relocation) were reported. Still, the point of the exercise was not to specifically uncover dramatic and life-shaping events but to identify events that typically signify important moments in life: graduation from school, marriage, the birth of children, employments, major events of illnesses and death within the family, retirement, and the like. Although the material was often prosaic, it inevitably happened that, in the recitation of the events of the decades, participants identified moments when some important attribute of the resident was first manifested, an attribute that would extend across the rest of the resident's life and would become one of the signature characteristics of the person. Whether this happened to be a strong allegiance to family, the love of travel, an artistic bent, or a personal trait such as humor, this time line exercise often proved to be the starting point for the identification and development of a theme that would be important in representing the resident to others through story.

Story Crafting

Whereas the first phase of the workshop concentrated on acquiring and ordering the facts of the resident's life, the second phase focused on identifying the resident's essence or character and on beginning to represent that character in narrative. Several elements contributed to address these aims; two of these elements were somewhat instructional in nature, and three others continued the process of involving the family members in giving shape to their ongoing research into their relative's life.

Two small instructional exercises were designed to provide family members with a framework and method for constructing their stories. In the first of these exercises, participants were asked to articulate, inductively, what they saw as the key elements of stories—in effect, they were asked to identify what they saw as the most common elements in stories they knew, novels they had read, or dramas they had seen in whatever medium. Although this was conducted as a brainstorming exercise, the facilitators did have a list in mind and were prepared, if necessary (and sometimes it was), to complete the list if participants did not come up with everything on it. The principal aim of this exercise was to make family members aware, as they began constructing their stories, that stories typically turn around a central problem or challenge and that character is usually revealed by how the central character faces and solves a problem or meets a challenge. At the same time, the facilitators sought, through the exercise, to strengthen family members' awareness that other elements are vital both to the meaning and to the delight that listeners take from stories. In that regard, the facilitators emphasized that elements such as scene setting, description, and mood or tone provide important shape to stories and that the management of time or sequence contributes mightily to the clarity of the story.

The second instructional exercise focused on the use of storyboards in the development of stories. The aim of the exercise was to help family members to understand that stories typically develop in scenes and that, in the most typical of narrative structures, the scenes usually proceed in a relatively fixed sequence: introduction of characters, introduction of a conflict or problem, crisis, and resolution. Comic strips were used as the main prop for this exercise. Virtually every participant in our study was familiar with at least one comic strip, so the exercise required little introduction. Both daily and Sunday comics were used to illustrate the point that many comic strips introduce and solve problems in a single strip (the characters usually are known). What was most helpful about this exercise was that it provided family members with a structure for the work of sketching out the stories they would tell. It helped them to think about their stories in terms of a string of frames and to realize that there had to be a clear enough story line so that the listener or viewer could understand how the frames were connected. The more sophisticated participants could also appreciate how illustration helped to create both scene and mood.

The three exercises that extended the process of fact gathering into a process of character identification involved family members in

1. Portraying the resident's life in developmental terms

2. Identifying abstract nouns that could describe key themes of the resident's life or key elements of his or her character

3. Selecting representations of the resident

In the first of these, family members were instructed to recast the decade-by-decade time line they had constructed into a more fluid representation of their relative's life, one organized by occurrences (e.g., events, decisions, changes) that reflected his or her development or maturation; these were meant to be the shaping events of the person's life. The criterion for selection of such events was the influence they had in the resident's life: the way in which they shaped future events, contributed to the character of the resident, or served to represent, in some essential fashion, something fundamentally true about who the resident was. These moments were as varied as the residents whose stories were being told: the first train trip as a young girl of a woman whose life was to be characterized by a sense of adventure and daring; the dutiful and willing walking home through the rain of a young man—at the instruction of his sweetheart, later his wife—the center of whose life would be his devotion to this woman who now had dementia; the first needlepoint creations made by a girl whose later life would always include an appreciation for art and artistry; the early death of a sibling of a woman whose life would be centered fiercely on her family; and reckless adolescent activities by a woman who would go on to be an overprotective mother. As family members began to plot their relatives' lives on a shaping-events backdrop, they began to describe their relatives more in terms of who they were than what they did. Asking them to see facts through the lens of development seemed to allow them to compress time so that they could use life events as a way to describe character. In storyboarding terms, the developmental history exercise gave participants a way to look at events and reveal something fundamental about the resident and to end their recounting of these events with a last frame that, in effect, indicated the element of character that the particular event illustrated, revealed, or foreshadowed.

In the second of these story-crafting exercises, the facilitators provided participants with a long list of abstract terms (e.g., family, work, religion, art, food, travel, service, money) and general characteristics (e.g., generous, vain, selfish, giving) and asked them to consider their relative in such terms—or others they might add to the list. This exercise was intended to reinforce the emphasis of this section of the workshop on getting at the essence or character of the resident and on structuring stories in a way that represented and illuminated this core. The exercise was somewhat redundant for many participants. They had already begun to describe their relative in general, characterizing terms—artist, scholar, prankster, mother, and so forth. However, because the workshops involved people from a wide variety of backgrounds, for some participants this exercise was helpful. It provided them with a way to organize into one or two general themes the elements of the life that they were seeing as somehow resonant of their relative.

The final story-crafting exercise engaged participants in a kind of scavenger hunt to find tangible, nonverbal ways to represent the resident to the audience for whom they were preparing their stories. Originally, the instructions for this exercise were to search through old photo albums and to bring in a collection of photos that each participant felt showed something important or revealing about the resident. In this original form, the facilitators asked participants to break into groups of two or three and to use the small group as a vehicle for narrating the individual pictures and for selecting a smaller set that they would then narrate to the large group. The idea was both to use the photos as props in developing small stories or frames in stories and to get used to the idea of editing material to achieve economy in storytelling. This exercise proved to be very powerful on a number of levels. For many participants, reviewing the visual history proved to be more emotionally powerful than dealing with facts and themes. The life of the person, often captured in high moments, was spread out for the family member, and, in some fashion, the family member's grief seemed to be triggered or unleashed by the exercise. For some participants, it was only through looking at the photos that everything clicked into focus about their relative. The most dramatic example of this was the case of a niece who had, throughout the workshop, described her aunt in relatively negative terms (e.g., selfish, self-centered, stingy, vain). While going through the photos, this niece had found a photo of her aunt as a young woman. Seeing how strikingly beautiful the aunt had been provided the niece with an epiphany: This was a woman virtually cursed by beauty—she was a person who had been pushed to live up to the admiration that others projected on her but could not. Through this sudden insight, the niece began to see the aunt in a different light, as someone who had always had to struggle to preserve something of herself while being forced to please others. Nor was this an isolated case. The images hit many family members on a different emotional and perceptual plane, and they saw and understood things about their relatives that were different from but complementary to what they had been seeing through the vehicle of narrative.

It was workshop participants themselves who broke past the equation that the workshops had established between representations and photos and began to use other media to invoke the spirit of the resident. A mounted version of a successful invention, paintings, a quilt—family members settled on these and other objects (instead of or in addition to photos) as ways to bring the character of their relative into focus. In one case, a family member created a French buffet for the group to recall the resident's (a former high school teacher) love of the culture and creativity of the French.

Performance Shaping

By the time family members had reached the point of identifying life themes and selecting representations, they had begun to speak about their relative in terms of stories. Earlier parts of the fact-gathering process had led them to select nodal points in their relative's life, and the explicit focus on narrative precipitated by the exercises dedicated to story elements and storyboarding established a kind of storytelling convention within the group. By the time they were about two thirds through the workshop, most participants had established a small repertoire of key and illuminating moments in the life of their relative and had begun to recount these in narrative (story) form. In this final phase of the workshop, the group itself played an important role in aiding its members through the final steps of preparation, selection, editing, and rehearsing.

The assignment given to participants for the second-to-last meeting of the group was to present to the group the list of small stories they planned to present to the care staff. This was not a surprise. Throughout the workshop, the facilitators and family members typically indicated when they felt a particular moment or incident was important and should be included in the presentation to staff. Although the final decision about this list was clearly that of the family member, the facilitators found that the group was not hesitant about providing input in this late session, especially if the family member had left out what the group considered to be an essential vignette. A number of final lists underwent significant change as a result of this session.

In the remainder of this session and throughout the final session of the workshop, family members practiced their story in front of the group. Because so much bonding had occurred during the course of the workshop, this was a comfortable setting for rehearsal, even for participants who had little experience performing in front of a group and who demonstrated clear signs of stage fright. The reinforcing ethos of this session always seemed to come naturally to the group and always seemed to provide family members with a boost in confidence for their upcoming performance before the staff. At the same time, this session gave the group a last chance to provide feedback and editorial comment. Comments at this stage were primarily meant to refine rather than reshape the final version to be presented to staff. However, in more than one instance, the group continued to insist on the inclusion of material that the family member still had not put into the narrative. One wife, for example, had captured the romance of the couple's courtship and early marriage (thereby portraying something very important about the husband's loving nature) but had—to the group's mind, at least—not sufficiently captured his passion for learning and his successes in his academic career. In the second-to-last session, the group had asked her to include this material; when it did not show up in her rehearsal performance, they again urged its inclusion, and, indeed, it was provided in the staff presentation.

Story presentations varied greatly and in a number of ways, but the two main variables were the style of presentation and the size and composition of the audience. Family members' own levels of comfort and experience shaped their presentations. Those who were practiced and comfortable in front of groups appeared at ease and spoke from memory or from notes. Those unaccustomed to public speaking wrote out what they wanted to share and read from their text. In one case, a woman who knew she would be very uncomfortable had herself videotaped beforehand and was present for questions when the tape was played to the staff. In our experience, both kinds of presentations were very well received. There was genuine appreciation for the gift of the stories and for the labor that had gone into crafting them.

The field test of the program was conducted in several nursing homes, and the level of commitment to and enthusiasm for the program by the organization was the principal determinant of staff attendance. In some cases, large groups of care staff were present; in other cases only a few were able to be freed from work to attend. During the field trial, the authors of this chapter were able to videotape the presentations, and these tapes were made available to the facilities so that any staff member could watch them.

RESULTS AND LESSONS LEARNED

As previously reported (Caron et al., 1999; Hepburn et al., 1997), the main finding of the field test of the Family Stories Workshop was that virtually all participants "got it." That is, participants caught on to the basic idea that they had something important to share with the care staff and that sharing through storytelling could be a very effective way to do so. All family members appreciated that there was an essence or core to their relative and that it would be good for the care staff to know something of that. Most participants came to understand the difference between listing facts and accomplishments and selecting and shaping them into a set of stories. Practically everyone who began the workshop completed it, and practically everyone did arrange for and make a presentation at a staff gathering. The majority of participants put together a presentation that reached the level of story (rather than list).

The workshops drew a wide variety of participants. Educational levels were much more divergent than the authors of this chapter had expected; those with some high school education mixed easily with those with graduate training. The groups were strikingly intergenerational: spouses and adult children were present in roughly equal numbers, but grandchildren and a grandniece showed up as well.

The process seemed to have a positive effect on participants in a number of ways. Perhaps the most significant effect of the workshop on participants was the manner in which it enabled them to step away from a disease-saturated discourse regarding the resident and to embrace a discourse that was more affirming and accepting (Caron et al., 1999). The participants were used to talking about the resident in terms of his or her illness and decline, but the workshop allowed family members to revisit the resident's whole life and to speak of the resident in terms of the challenges he or she faced and the accomplishments of that life. This seemed to lead some to a recovery or rebalancing that appeared to be very satisfying. Another positive effect that occurred in several cases was that the process of developing the stories enabled participants to identify and resolve conflicts they had about their relative. The son who came to understand the other side of his mother's protectiveness and controlling behavior and the niece who saw behind her aunt's vanity serve as examples of the kind of resolution that occurred in several instances. In some cases, the process helped to draw families together. The dementing disorder, family members' appraisal of the disorder and its effects, and the caregiving process, so typically involving just one family member as principal caregiver, can create or exacerbate divisions in families. In some cases, when the family member drew others into the story-building process (either to gather facts or to help develop the stories), the process served to restore some cohesion to these families.

The workshops occasionally had secondary social effects on participants. In many cases, genuine fondness developed among group members, so participation appeared to have a salutary effect: People had fun in the groups. In a number of cases, participants connected with each other outside of the group, primarily by phone and largely to provide support or information linked to their continuing role as caregivers. In one exceptional case, a number of members of one of the workshop groups formed a social club that continued to meet on a regular basis long after the workshop was over. The performance events also provided a setting for positive social interactions. For most of the performances, other members of the storytellers' families were present; in several cases, other family members offered spontaneous recountings of vignettes that were in the spirit of the main storyteller's narrative.

One of the most consistent experiences of the workshops was the questioning by family members about their responsibility toward the story subject regarding the confidentiality of information. How explicit were the stories to be, and how much personal information could family members provide to others? One participant wondered whether she needed her relative's informed consent to share his story. The facilitators' suggestion to groups was that they could see themselves as standing surrogate for the resident. Within this construction, the facilitators suggested that they ask themselves: If he or she were telling the story, what would he or she include and what would he or she leave out based on what you understand about his or her level of comfort with self-disclosure? The group also discussed poetic license. That is, the facilitators made it clear to family members that embellishment within the broad limits of the facts of the story would not be inappropriate in the service of emphasizing the point of the story.

Reports of the impact of the stories on staff during the field trial were anecdotal in nature. There was universal appreciation for the effort that family members made in developing the stories and an equal degree of enthusiasm for the presentations themselves. Staff seemed to grasp not only how much "work" it took to put the stories together but also how intensely meaningful the stories were for family members, and there was a high level of appreciation for the meaningfulness of the activity and the event. There was a clear sense that a gift had been given. The Family Stories Workshop had occasional reports that the stories provided insight into the resident in ways that influenced care. The best example came from reports from staff members that the family presentation helped them understand that the quirky behaviors of an imposing resident might not be menacing but rather might reflect a long history of playful provocation; in short, they became less afraid of the resident.

CONCLUSION

Our experience with the Family Stories Workshop was brief, limited by the terms of the field trial. The trial demonstrated the considerable power of the story and the great, untapped reservoir of stories and storytelling that resides in families. Clearly, within the limits of the experiment, the process and the families intersected in ways that produced lovely stories and satisfying involvement for the families and care staff. It was also clear that the material delivered in the stories went far beyond the kind of information that is typically included in the social history section of admitting assessments: Spirit exceeds—but also vivifies—fact.

Institutions providing care for individuals with dementing disorders could readily implement the Family Stories Workshop, but there are several requirements or preconditions:

- *The groups need facilitators.* Even though group members played an increasingly important role in the process as the group moved through its stages, it is unlikely the workshop could be run as a self-directed group. Someone has to maintain the agenda, make brief presentations, assure that members participate, and interface with the organization to arrange for story presentations. As noted, the authors of this chapter found staff members in a number of capacities who came to serve as cofacilitators, so it is evident there are skills available to meet the task. The authors of this chapter also believe that volunteer family members—perhaps "graduates" of the program—could facilitate the groups.

- *Staff time for attendance has to be assured.* The clearest expression of the organization's commitment to the importance of the program (in addition to providing cookies and coffee for the sessions) is its willingness to enable care staff to attend the presentation of stories. This involves an investment. If staff members are to attend during work time, the facility has to pay them. The authors of this chapter believe that this is an investment by the facility, one that expresses its belief in the importance of person-centered care and that endorses the importance of a developed partnership between staff and families, one based in a sensitive appreciation for the resident who cannot recount his or her own story.

- *A method of incorporating the material needs to be found.* In many cases, the material embodied in the stories sheds important light on who the resident was and is, information that could bear importantly on the staff's assessment and care plan. At the very least, facilities hosting the Family Stories Workshop should avail themselves of the opportunities the stories provide to allow care provision to be influenced by the stories. Second, the commitment by the family member to develop and share the story represents a serious offer of partnership. Facilities should find ways to work meaningfully with these family members in the ongoing care of the resident.

The Family Stories Workshop is a modest activity that demonstrated considerably positive results. With a modest investment, organizations could implement such workshops. The workshops do not resolve all of the issues and tensions that can exist between families and staff, but they do seem to provide a generous common meeting place where new and positive relationships can develop, relationships that can benefit family, staff, and, most important, the person who cannot tell his or her own tale.

REFERENCES

Alzheimer's Association. (2004). Statistics about Alzheimer's disease. Retrieved September 15, 2004, from http://www.alz.org/AboutAD/statistics.asp

Aneshensel, C.S., Pearlin, L.I., Mullan, J.T., Zarit, S.H., & Whitlatch, C.J. (1995). *Profiles in caregiving: The unexpected career.* San Diego: Academic Press.

Caron, W., Hepburn, K., Luptak, M., Grant, L., Ostwald, S., & Keenan, J. (1999). Expanding the discourse of care: Family constructed biographies of nursing home residents. *Families, Systems, & Health, 17,* 323–335.

Heiselman, T., & Noelker, L. (1991). Enhancing mutual respect among nursing assistants, residents, and residents' families. *The Gerontologist, 31,* 552–555.

Hepburn, K.W., Caron, W., Luptak, M., Ostwald, S., Grant, L., & Keenan, J.M. (1997). The Families Stories Workshop: Stories for those who cannot remember. *The Gerontologist, 37,* 827–832.

Magaziner, J., German, P., Zimmerman, S.I., Hebel, J.R., Burton, L., Gruber-Baldini, A.L., et al. (2000). The prevalence of dementia in a statewide sample of new nursing home admissions age 65 and over: Diagnosis by expert panel. *The Gerontologist, 40,* 663–672.

Pinquart, M., & Sorensen, S. (2003a). Associations of stressors and uplifts of caregiving with caregiver burden and depressive mood: A meta-analysis.

Journals of Gerontology. Series B, Psychological Sciences and Social Sciences, 58, P112–P128.

Pinquart, M., & Sorensen, S. (2003b). Differences between caregivers and noncaregivers in psychological health and physical health: A meta-analysis. *Psychology and Aging, 18,* 250–267.

Rubin, A., & Shuttlesworth, G.E. (1983). Engaging families as support resources in nursing home care: Ambiguity in the subdivision of tasks. *The Gerontologist, 23,* 632–636.

Schulz, R., Belle, S.H., Czaja, S.J., McGinnis, K.A., Stevens, A., & Zhang, S. (2004). Long-term care placement of dementia patients and caregiver health and well-being. *JAMA, 292,* 961–967.

Schwarz, A.N., & Vogel, M.E. (1990). Nursing home staff and residents' families role expectations. *The Gerontologist, 30,* 169–183.

Shuttlesworth, G.E., Rubin, A., & Duffy, M. (1982). Families versus institutions: Incongruent role expectations in the nursing home. *The Gerontologist, 22,* 200–208.

Sumaya-Smith, I. (1995). Caregiver/resident relationships: Surrogate family bonds and surrogate grieving in a skilled nursing facility. *Journal of Advanced Nursing, 21,* 446–451.

Tornatore, J.B., & Grant, L.A. (2002). Burden among family caregivers of persons with Alzheimer's disease in nursing homes. *The Gerontologist, 42,* 497–506.

Vitaliano, P.P., Zhang, J., & Scanlan, J.M. (2003). Is caregiving hazardous to one's physical health? A meta-analysis. *Psychological Bulletin, 129,* 946–972.

RESOURCES

For information about the Family Stories Workshop as well as comments and questions about its design, implementation, and evaluation, please contact

Kenneth Hepburn, Ph.D.
Professor and Associate Dean for Research
University of Minnesota
School of Nursing
6-169 Weaver-Densford Hall
308 Harvard Street SE
Minneapolis, MN 55455
E-mail: hepbu001@umn.edu
Telephone: 612-625-1678

Wayne A. Caron, Ph.D.
Lecturer
Department of Family Social Science

University of Minnesota
290 McNeal Hall
1985 Buford Avenue
St Paul, MN 55108
E-mail: wcaron@umn.edu
Telephone: 612-625-1900

8

Family Involvement in the Care of Residents with Dementia

An Important Resource for Quality of Life and Care

JANET K. PRINGLE SPECHT, DAVID REED, AND MERIDEAN L. MAAS

Mr. Tomas, a 70-year-old retired accountant, has lived in a nursing home for 6 months. His wife admitted him after taking care of him at home for 5 years. After he had gotten outdoors and wandered away repeatedly, she decided she could no longer maintain him safely at home. She admitted him with some trepidation because she was not sure he would get satisfactory care at the nursing home, even though she knew the facility had a good reputation. The thought of turning his care over to someone else was very worrisome and made her quite anxious. Because Mr. and Mrs. Tomas lived in a community some distance from the nursing home, Mrs. Tomas rented an apartment in the town where the nursing home is located. This removed Mrs. Tomas from the support she usually received from friends and her church family.

Mrs. Prin is a 66-year-old widow with mid-stage dementia. She was admitted to the nursing home a year ago when she was no longer able to care for herself at home without constant supervision. Mrs. Prin has three daughters, but only one, Doris, lives in the area. Doris is very attentive but is extremely busy with her job and family responsibilities. She usually visits once every week or two. She talks often about how guilty she feels about putting her mother in a home and not visiting her more often.

These two examples represent the difficulties that family members often encounter when an elderly relative has dementia. Family members of people with dementia often suffer great physical, emotional, and social strain in their lives. Dementia, a common and devastating health problem, affects 8%–10% of individuals age 65 and older and more than 30% of individuals older than 85. Approximately 4 to 6 million people in the United States have one of several types of dementia (Unverzagt et al., 2001). Although the most prevalent types are Alzheimer's disease and vascular dementia, and there are variations in the speed and manifestations of decline in all types of dementia, all share a similar deteriorating course including memory loss, confusion, language difficulties, and eventually the loss of physical functioning. These manifestations affect both the person with the disease and the family members who love and care for him or her (Volicer, McKee, & Hewitt, 2001). As a result, the stress of family caregiving is a health care concern that has generated substantial research (Goode, Haley, Roth, & Ford, 1998; Pinquart & Sorensen, 2003a, 2003b; Vitaliano, Zhang, & Scanlan, 2003; Wilcox & King, 1999; Wright, Clipp, & George, 1993). However, most of this research covers the period when the person with dementia is cared for at home (Acton & Kang, 2001; Chang, 1999; Ostwald, Hepburn, Caron, Burns, & Mantell, 1999; Wilkens, Castle, Heck, Tanzy, & Fahey, 1999). Some more recent studies are documenting the effects of family caregiving stress following the admission of a relative with dementia to residential care (Canadian Study of Health and Aging Working Group, 2002; Gaugler, Pearlin, Leitsch, & Davey, 2001; Gaugler, Zarit, & Pearlin, 2003; Grant et al., 2002; Tornatore & Grant, 2002).

Relocation of a relative to a nursing home in the later stages of dementia is common (Hagen, 2001), resulting in approximately 60% of nursing home residents reported to be persons with dementia (Magaziner et al., 2000). Relocation relieves many problems for family caregivers, but it does not necessarily mean an end to their caregiving or stress (Bauer & Nay, 2003; Dellasega & Mastrian, 1995; Hagen, 2001). Family caregiver stress often continues and may even be exacerbated. Family caregiving following relocation has received less attention; however, reports of several studies indicate that families remain involved in their relatives' care (Bowers, 1988; Duncan & Morgan, 1994; Friedemann, Montgomery, Rice, & Farrell, 1999; Gaugler, Anderson, Zarit, & Pearlin, 2004; Gaugler et al., 2003; Kelley, Swanson, Maas, & Tripp-Reimer, 1999; Moss, Lawton, Kleban, & Duhamel, 1993).

Following relocation, family caregivers must develop a different role in the care of their relatives (Connell, Janevic, & Gallant, 2001; Kellett, 1998). Many caregivers must adjust their role from total responsibility to nearly complete exclusion from caregiving, yet they feel obliged to continue caregiving (Butcher, Holkup, Park, & Maas, 2001). Thus, the stress of caregiving may increase as a result of loss of control of caregiving, a less intimate relationship with the care recipient, guilt from moving the care recipient to a nursing home, feelings of confinement resulting from the obligation to provide or oversee care, and conflict with staff caregivers, who often view family members as visitors who should not be involved with the care of the resident with dementia (Bauer & Nay, 2003).

Relocation of the relative can offer family caregivers opportunities not previously available (Fink & Picot, 1995). With the potential cessation of direct, hands-on care responsibilities following relocation, family members can have more time available to devote to the relationship and to enhancing the relative's quality of life. Unfortunately, family members usually are uncertain about how to shift from a direct caregiving role to a more indirect, supportive interpersonal role, and they may receive little or no assistance from nursing home staff when doing so (Kelley, Swanson, et al., 1999; Montgomery & Montoro, 1995). Friedemann, Montgomery, Maiberger, and Smith (1997) reported that staff members overlooked and ignored families who tried to give them advice or treated family members insensitively.

In nursing homes, staff members struggle with the demands and stress of caring for people with dementia, a task typically made more difficult by understaffing, high turnover, minimal training, and limited professional nurse leadership. Once a resident is admitted to a nursing home, staff members may not be open to family member participation in care. Institutional staff members have traditionally planned care and assumed the primary role of ensuring that agency goals are met and quality care is delivered (Specht et al., 2000). It is not unusual for nursing home staff to advise family members that they should not visit their relative for 2–3 weeks after admission so that the relative will "become adjusted." The staff may assure family members that care staff members now have primary responsibility for the resident. This marks the transition of a family member from the role of caregiver to that of visitor and shifts control of care from the family and even the care recipient to the staff.

Family members' requests and attempts to help care for their relatives are often viewed by staff members as interruptions that add to the burden and stress of their work. Staff members have variously been encouraged to view the resident's family members as clients (Hall & Buckwalter, 1987; Montgomery, 1982), as a needed resource for care (Montgomery, 1982; Spencer, 1991), or as partners in care (Maas,

Buckwalter, Swanson, Specht, et al., 1994; Spencer, 1991; Travis, 1996), but staff and family members report difficulties in sharing their caregiving roles or adequately specifying who has responsibility for particular care tasks (Bonder, 1986; Bowers, 1988; Rubin & Shuttlesworth, 1983; Maas et al., 2004). Unfortunately, the staff's view of "client" is too often of another person with needs who must be cared for rather than as someone who has needs but who participates in problem solving and maintains control of decisions (Friedemann et al., 1999). As Montgomery (1982) warned, the view of family members as staff helpers and merely a resource (family as servant) fails to support high-quality family and staff relations or the maintenance of the involvement of family members in the life of their relative. Family–staff role conflicts are stressful for staff members as well as families, depriving them of the benefits of cooperation, personal information about residents, and coordination of caregiving efforts (Maas et al., 1992). These circumstances underscore the need for an intervention to assist family and staff caregivers to form a partnership in the care of a person with dementia who is relocated to a nursing home.

The experiences of Mr. Tomas and Mrs. Prin provide real-life examples of how family and staff relationships often become strained and conflicted because of the lack of purposeful efforts to form cooperative family and staff role expectations and to involve family members in the care of their relatives as partners with staff caregivers.

After Mr. Tomas is admitted to the nursing home, Mrs. Tomas visits daily, usually spending 4-6 hours each day on the unit with her husband. Mr. Tomas is still able to walk, although he stumbles easily, putting him at high risk for falls. He communicates very little verbally and needs assistance with all of his activities of daily living. He is beginning to have some swallowing difficulties. Mrs. Tomas has many complaints about the care. Staff members dread seeing her arrive in the morning and usually try to avoid her by not going into Mr. Tomas's room when she is visiting. She often makes cutting remarks to the staff, such as "Could you turn Jake now, or are you too busy going on break?" or "You would think any simpleton could remember to wash his face after you help him with breakfast!" Mr. Tomas's appearance and his meals are of special concern to her. She relates that he had always been very meticulous about his appearance and really enjoyed his food. "Food is one of the few pleasures he has left," she often tells the staff.

The nursing staff is very concerned about Mrs. Prin, who has few visitors, does not participate in any activities, and often cries. The staff members cannot understand why her daughter, Doris, who lives nearby, doesn't visit more often and why, when she does, she seldom stays more than 15 minutes. They feel sorry for Mrs. Prin and hope that their own families will treat them better if they ever have to live in a nursing home. Staff members believe that Mrs. Prin would be happier and cry less if the daughter was more attentive, but they know very little about Mrs. Prin or her daughter.

The small but increasing body of literature on family involvement following nursing home placement has shown that the level and type of family involvement in the care of a relative in a nursing home are related to family satisfaction, family stress, and resident adjustment (Friedemann et al., 1997; Ryan & Scullion, 2000; also see the introductory chapter in this book). This chapter describes the rationale and theoretical framework for the Family Involvement in Care (FIC) intervention that was tested in nursing home dementia special care units (SCUs). Following a detailed description of the FIC intervention, specific guidelines for implementation are presented. Findings of the study that tested the outcome effects of the FIC intervention for family members and SCU staff are discussed. Additional findings for families and staff are reported elsewhere (Butcher et al., 2001; Jablonski, Reed, & Maas, 2005; Kelley, Swanson, et al., 1999; Maas et al., 1992). Case examples (Mr. Tomas and Mrs. Prin) are also provided to illustrate implementation of the FIC intervention, including the negotiation of a family–staff partnership plan. Finally, practice and research implications of the study's findings are presented.

THEORETICAL FRAMEWORK

Theoretical models of person–environment fit and interaction (Kahana, 1982; Lawton, 1982; Parr, 1980), the Progressively Lowered Stress Threshold model (Hall & Buckwalter, 1987), and role theory (Hardy & Conway, 1978; O'Neill & Ross, 1991) support the FIC intervention. Figure 8.1 depicts the relationships among major concepts and the hypothesized family and staff outcome effects of the FIC intervention.

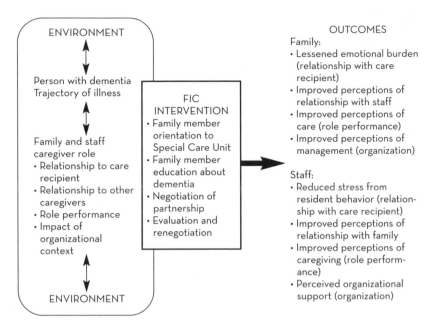

ENVIRONMENT

Person with dementia
Trajectory of illness

Family and staff
caregiver role
• Relationship to care
  recipient
• Relationship to other
  caregivers
• Role performance
• Impact of
  organizational
  context

ENVIRONMENT

FIC
INTERVENTION
• Family member
  orientation to
  Special Care Unit
• Family member
  education about
  dementia
• Negotiation of
  partnership
• Evaluation and
  renegotiation

OUTCOMES
Family:
• Lessened emotional burden
  (relationship with care
  recipient)
• Improved perceptions of
  relationship with staff
• Improved perceptions of
  care (role performance)
• Improved perceptions of
  management (organization)

Staff:
• Reduced stress from
  resident behavior (relationship with care recipient)
• Improved perceptions of
  relationship with family
• Improved perceptions of
  caregiving (role performance)
• Perceived organizational
  support (organization)

Figure 8.1.   Theoretical framework for Family Involvement in Care (FIC) intervention and outcomes.

Person–environment fit and interaction are conceptualized along a trajectory of changes over time for residents with dementia, family members, and staff caregivers. In addition to guiding awareness of the
increasingly compromised abilities of people with dementia to cope
with environmental cues and stimuli, the theoretical framework assists
with understanding the role-related stressors for family and staff caregivers and suggests interventions to relieve the stress and increase
positive attitudes.

Listed in Table 8.1 are four fundamental aspects of the caregiving
role. For both family and staff members in the SCU setting, these include
the caregiver relationship to the care recipient, the relationship between
family and staff caregivers, adequacy of role performance (adequacy
of care), and the organizational context. The expectation formed by
the theoretical framework is that intervening to improve the fit of
family and staff caregiving roles and relationships will improve caregiver outcomes. The specific intervention designed to improve the fit
is the FIC protocol for negotiated partnerships between family and
staff caregivers. This intervention directly influences one aspect of the
caregiving role (creating a new relationship between family and staff

Table 8.1. Clusters of outcome measurement scales in relation to aspects of caregiving role for family and staff caregivers

	Character of the outcome cluster scales in each cluster			
Aspects of Caregiving Role	Family	alpha	Staff	alpha
Relationships to care recipient	Emotional reactions to care recipient		Emotional reactions to care recipient's	
	Loss	.73	Inappropriate behavior	.94
	Captivity	.81	Aggress on	.94
	Guilt	.70		
Relationship to other caregivers	Perceived relationship with staff		Perceived relationship with family	
	Conflict	.84	Dominion	.71
	Disregard	.85	Exclusion	.70
			Disruption	.64
			Partnership	.58
			Irrelevance	.60
Adequacy of role performance	Perceptions of care		Perception of caregiving	
	Physical care	.97	Role inadequacy	.82
	Activities	.87	Task burden	.84
			Resident harm	.83
Impact of organizational context	Perceptions of management effectiveness		Perceived organizational support	
	Management	.88	Resources	.81

Key: alpha = reliability score.

169

caregivers), and it was expected that this new relationship would make it possible for other aspects of family and staff caregiving roles to be redefined as well. That is, relationships to the care recipient are also redefined, and the quality of care provided by both types of caregiver is enhanced. Further details of the theoretical framework and its relationship to the intervention can be found in Maas, Buckwalter, Swanson, Specht, et al. (1994).

THE FIC INTERVENTION

The FIC intervention develops partnerships between family caregiver(s) and long-term care facility staff in order to provide the best possible care for a resident with dementia. An underlying assumption of the FIC intervention is that both parties must continually negotiate and clarify their expectations to establish mutually satisfactory roles and relationships. Another key assumption is that the staff will help family members choose the type and frequency of care activities in which each family member wants to participate without any coercion to participate in more activities than the family member desires.

The FIC intervention protocol is composed of four key elements:

1. Orientation of an identified primary family caregiver (and other family caregivers, if they wish to participate) to the facility, the SCU, and the proposed partnership role

2. Education of family members for involvement in the care of a person with dementia

3. Negotiation and formation of a partnership agreement

4. A follow-up with family members and staff to evaluate and renegotiate the partnership agreement (Maas, Buckwalter, Swanson, Specht, et al., 1994)

Orientation and Advance Preparation

Prior to implementing the FIC, SCU staff caregivers receive education about the rationale for the FIC intervention and its advantages for family members and staff caregivers, including how the care of residents with dementia is enhanced.

A family–staff conference for negotiating the partnership and the form and extent of family member involvement in care is central to

Table 8.2. Orientation and preparation phase

1.	Gather information about the resident and family from the resident's record, the resident, the family, and other staff members.
2.	Elicit support of all staff for the partnership; involve caregiving staff as much as possible in planning and implementing the partnership.
3.	Identify needs of the resident with which the family caregiver could potentially assist.
4.	Share information on activities and partnerships with family members.
5.	Contact the family to encourage family participation, questions, comments, and so forth.
6.	Schedule a mutually convenient/appropriate time and location for the partnership negotiation.

the intervention. The activities, intensity of participation, contact length, and frequency of contact are negotiated, agreed upon, and documented on a partnership agreement form (see Chapter 8 Appendix).

The purpose of the orientation and preparation phase (see Table 8.2) is to establish a foundation for the FIC intervention. There are three important steps in this phase:

1. A formal care provider who will act as the liaison with the family member is identified (a nurse care manager is particularly helpful because of the primacy of nursing care).

2. The staff liaison visits with the family member to identify primary family caregivers.

3. The family caregiver is taken on a tour of the care environment, and the liaison reviews philosophies and policies and discusses expectations and concerns.

This orientation and preparation phase includes negotiating a partnership agreement for the involvement of families in the care of relatives with dementia. The partnership negotiation meeting is described next and is illustrated through case studies.

Staff Training and Family Education

Eight hours of training delivered in three sessions prepared staff members in the experimental sites for negotiating sessions with family caregivers. The first session presented information about dementia and its impact on residents, family, and staff and was provided to staff members in both experimental and control sites following baseline data collection. The second session, presented only to the staff at experimental sites, emphasized the problems faced by family members of residents in a long-term care facility, oriented staff to the FIC intervention and its rationale, and used case studies and role playing for staff members to practice its implementation. All nursing staff members working on the experimental units were expected to attend the first two sessions. A third session stressed how to negotiate the role family members could assume in providing care. Only staff members who negotiated agreements with family members were required to attend the third session. Personnel hired after the initial training sessions either received a repeat of the original sessions or completed a self-study module. Objectives for each session of the staff training are included in the Appendix.

Education of the family caregiver began with a manual created by the investigators, the FIC Educational Resource Manual. The manual contains activities and interventions designed for people with dementia. Selected categories of these activities and interventions are art therapy, approaches for relating with the resident and managing behaviors, environmental structuring, exercise, eating and nutrition, medication management, music therapy, strategies to avoid physical restraint, personal care, and therapeutic recreation. The primary nurse discussed with the family caregiver specific ways to make involvement in therapeutic activities and personal care meaningful and enjoyable for both the family caregiver and the resident. The guiding characteristics of successful partnerships were emphasized repeatedly in the training for the family members and staff caregivers (see Figure 8.2).

Partnership Negotiation Meetings

The process of negotiating the partnership agreement is described in detail in Table 8.3. Activities that families agreed to perform during the FIC study ranged from simple provision of information about the resident to active participation in physical care and assistance with psychosocial modalities (see Table 8.4).

Informed,
flexible,
common goals.
Agreement on roles
produces positive results,
based on mutual respect, and
negotiated power and involvement.

Figure 8.2.   Characteristics of successful family–staff partnerships.

Table 8.3. Partnership negotiation

1.	Set a nonthreatening tone.
2.	Welcome all participants to the meeting.
3.	Discuss the importance of staff and family in caring for the resident and making decisions about care.
4.	Discuss the common goal of achieving the best possible resident care.
5.	Acknowledge that family members and staff will likely have different perspectives about resident care.
6.	Encourage all participants to listen to each other.
7.	Commit to finding creative, mutually acceptable solutions to different perspectives.
8.	Encourage the family members to express their concerns about the resident, nursing home care, and their role in caregiving.
9.	Encourage staff and family members to express their thoughts/concerns about their respective roles, the residents, and the involvement of families in care.
10.	Discuss the current caregiving activities of the family members.
11.	Identify specific needs of the resident.
12.	Discuss activities that would meet these needs.
13.	Discuss activities in which the family members would like to be involved.
14.	Discuss the pros and cons of the family members' preferences for involvement.
15.	Negotiate changes in preferences if necessary.
16.	Identify staff activities needed to facilitate the family members' involvement.
17.	Describe the specific roles of staff and family members on the partnership agreement form (make copies for the facility record and the family).
18.	Thank the family members for participating, arrange a monthly schedule to contact them to see how things are going, and encourage family members contact with staff liaison for questions, concerns, or suggestions.

The cases of Mr. Tomas and Mrs. Prin further illustrate the negotiation of the FIC partnership agreement.

In the partnership meeting, Mrs. Tomas expressed her concern about the care not being what she would like it to be. She was particularly concerned about Mr. Tomas's grooming. Often when she arrived mid-morning, Mr. Tomas still had the remains of breakfast on his face, and sometimes his shirt was soiled. The staff expressed concern that Mrs. Tomas was rude to them and had unreasonable expectations. Mrs. Tomas responded that she didn't mean to be rude, she just wanted good care for her husband and she didn't know how to make that happen. Discussion of goals for Mr. Tomas evolved to an agreement that both Mrs. Tomas and the staff wanted the best possible care for Mr. Tomas. This relieved the tension and focused the conversation on mutual goals for Mr. Tomas. Mrs. Tomas and the staff agreed on the following goals:

1. Ensure that Mr. Tomas is well groomed, with particular attention following meals.

Table 8.4.   Family involvement in care activities

Family members construct a photo life storybook or room bulletin board.

  The photo life storybook can be used during visits.

  Family members share the life storybook with new staff.

  Staff members use the life storybook to reminisce with the resident on days when the family does not visit.

Family members supply the staff with information about the resident's life experience, personality, and accomplishments.

  Family members prepare an audiotape for all staff, containing descriptions.

  Family members participate in resident care conferences.

Family members assist with physical care (e.g., bathing, exercise, grooming).

  Wife assists with bathing on Monday and Thursday evenings.

  Daughter feeds her father lunch on Mondays, Wednesdays, and Fridays.

  Son trims his mother's fingernails every other week.

  Daughter-in-law monitors a resident's physical care by observing cleanliness of the resident and reporting any problems to a designated staff member.

Family members promote purposeful activity of a loved one.

  Wife accompanies her husband to church services on Sunday mornings.

  Daughter participates with her mother in craft sessions.

  Family members rotate turns coming to assist with the monthly unit activity.

---

2.   Maintain Mr. Tomas's ability to walk for as long as possible.

3.   Make mealtime a special time for Mr. Tomas, and provide him with foods he especially likes.

4.   Help Mr. Tomas have enjoyable days.

Responsibilities for Mrs. Tomas and the staff were delineated in a partnership agreement containing the specific activities agreed upon for staff and Mrs. Tomas in order to reach these goals (see Table 8.5).

Mrs. Prin's daughter, Doris, attended the negotiation meeting. She began the meeting by stating that she wanted the best for her mom and wanted to continue to be involved in her life. However, she said that her visits were very difficult because her mom just sat listlessly, looking at her hands and ignoring Doris's presence. She went on to say that their relationship had never been easy and now it seemed even worse. She said that she visited as often as she could but wished there was some way that her siblings at a distance could help. Staff reported that Mrs. Prin is very withdrawn most of the time, seldom leaves her room, and does not participate in any activities. Doris related that her mother was very accomplished with needlework, liked being with other people, and had had a wide range of interests.

Table 8.5.   Mr. Tomas's Partnership Agreement

Mrs. Tomas will

1. Help Mr. Tomas eat lunch each day during the week, washing his face and changing his shirt if needed after lunch.

2. Make and bring one of Mr. Tomas's favorite foods for lunch one time per month.

3. Accompany Mr. Tomas to one food-related activity monthly and help with the activity.

4. Report to the nurse each time she finds Mr. Tomas not well-groomed.

5. Take Mr. Tomas for a combined walk (Mr. Tomas will walk a longer distance each day or until tired) and wheelchair ride each afternoon.

6. Help Mr. Tomas plant tulip bulbs in the raised planter outside his window.

7. Meet with the staff and share information about Mr. Tomas and his life.

The staff will

1. Help Mr. Tomas with meals when Mrs. Tomas is not present and immediately wash his face, clean his dentures, and change his clothing if needed following meals. (assigned CNA)

2. Assure that Mr. Tomas is well-groomed (clean, dentures cleaned, hair combed, wearing matching clean clothing) before Mrs. Tomas arrives each day at 10:00 A.M. (CNA)

3. Arrange a meeting for Mrs. Tomas with the staff to share information about Mr. Tomas's life. Record the session for staff who cannot attend. (NCM)

4. Check with Mrs. Tomas each day for 1 week and then weekly to see if the care is satisfactory and report to the staff regarding concerns or satisfaction. (NCM)

5. Check at least hourly when Mrs. Tomas is visiting to see if anything is needed. (CNA)

6. Assist Mr. Tomas with a walk in the home each evening.

7. Arrange Mr. Tomas's participation and Mrs. Tomas's assistance with one food-related activity per month. (AT)

8. Set date for Mrs. Tomas to attend a conference with the staff to discuss progress with goals for Mr. Tomas and any needed renegotiation of the partnership. (NCM)

Key: AT, activity therapist; CNA, certified nursing assistant; NCM, nurse care manager.

The following mutual goals were established for Mrs. Prin's care and Doris's involvement:

1. Assess Mrs. Prin and intervene, if needed, for depression.

2. Involve Doris in Mrs. Prin's care by helping make the visits more pleasant for both the daughter and Mrs. Prin.

3. Involve the other siblings in Mrs. Prin's life.

4. Have staff learn more about Mrs. Prin's life so ways can be found to engage her in purposeful activities she would enjoy.

The partnership agreement for Mrs. Prin included the strategies to be used to meet the goals for Mrs. Prin and those to be implemented by the family member and staff (see Table 8.6).

The partnership implementation is the most important part of the intervention. It is essential for the staff liaison to share and discuss the

Table 8.6. Mrs. Prin's Partnership Agreement

Doris will

1. Meet with the staff and share information about Mrs. Prin's likes and dislikes, her interests, and her life.

2. Manicure Mrs. Prin's nails monthly as a way to promote personal contact and a sense of accomplishment.

3. Participate in decisions regarding the use of any psychotropic medications.

4. Contact her sisters to arrange with them to send cards and tapes that could be used by Doris and the staff for conversation and reminiscing with Mrs. Prin.

5. Bring a family album to look through with her mother.

6. Bring a simple needlework craft to see if Mrs. Prin is interested in working with it.

Staff will

1. Complete a depression assessment of Mrs. Prin and pursue treatment with the physician as needed. (NCM)

2. Keep Doris apprised of the findings of the assessment and the treatment plan. (NCM)

3. Arrange a staff meeting for Doris to talk about her mother. Record the session so staff unable to attend can also learn about Mrs. Prin. (NCM)

4. Check with Doris after each visit, share how the visit went, and discuss how to make it better, noting what was most effective. (NCM/SW)

5. Explore possible additional diversionary activities that Mrs. Prin would enjoy and plan for staff to provide the activities. (NCM & CNA)

6. Assure that equipment for nail care is available for Doris to do her mother's nails. (CNA)

7. Share with Doris what her mother says about the visits, when she is most responsive, and what goes on when Doris is not there. (CNA and NCM)

Key: CNA, certified nursing assistant; NCM, nurse care manager; SW, social worker.

agreed-upon partnership activities with staff members who were not able to attend the meeting. Arrangements also need to be made to provide the family with the training they may need to carry out the agreed-upon activities. Continuous feedback must be solicited from the staff about how the agreement is working and any suggestions they may have for improvement or modification.

Follow-Up Meetings

Renegotiation of the partnership agreement in monthly meetings is an important part of the intervention because it enables the adjustment of the agreement to the changing mental and physical condition of the residents and to family members' circumstances and the extent of involvement they want to continue. In addition, it enables family and staff members to discuss how the plan is working, modify the plan if needed, clarify any confusion, and pursue any problems encountered in the implementation.

At the end of 1 month, the relationship between Mrs. Tomas and the staff was much improved. Mrs. Tomas was much more satisfied with the care and was able to express her appreciation to staff members when she came and found Mr. Tomas impeccably groomed. The staff worked very hard to reach the mutual goals that were set and took on the challenge of providing excellent care. This improved relationship enabled staff members to be more supportive of Mrs. Tomas, who also was very lonely since moving to her apartment. A strong partnership resulted that helped them work together to meet the challenges that came as Mr. Tomas had increasing difficulty with swallowing and ambulation.

Assessment did show Mrs. Prin to be severely depressed, and the physician prescribed an antidepressant that lessened her listlessness and made her more accessible to interaction. Reminiscing with the use of the family album engaged Mrs. Prin and promoted sharing between her and her daughter, Doris, who thought the visits were going much better and increased her visits to weekly. Staff members were less judgmental and more supportive of Doris when she did visit. Staff shared happenings in Mrs. Prin's day-to-day life that helped Doris connect even more with her mother. Doris expressed that the relationship with her mother seemed improved. The daughters who lived out of town began sending cards monthly and sent tapes of their children playing the piano and singing. Doris and Mrs. Prin listened to these tapes together. Mrs. Prin still seldom left her room and did not participate in activities. The plan was modified to arrange for Doris to accompany her mother to an activity that would be particularly appealing based on her mother's previous interests. The activity staff agreed to use the information that Doris provided in her meeting with the staff to make a life storybook that staff members could use in reminiscing with Mrs. Prin at least three times per week.

Expected Outcomes

Examples of desired family caregivers' outcomes include decreased feelings of loss, guilt, and captivity (from obligations to provide care), which are associated with role stress in caregivers' relationships with the care recipient. Another positive outcome is the improvement of relationships with staff, particularly perceptions of conflict. Family members' satisfaction with the care received by their relatives should be more positive when family and staff members form effective caregiving partnerships. Likewise, staff members who are partners with family caregivers are expected to perceive their relationships with families in more positive ways. The partnerships also should relieve some stress of the task burden and role inadequacy perceived by facility staff, who often have limited personnel and knowledge resources to deal or interact with people with dementia and their family members (Maas, Buckwalter, Swanson, & Mobily, 1994; Maas & Swanson, 1992).

DESIGN AND METHODS OF THE FIC STUDY

Guided by the theoretical frameworks discussed in the previous section, outcomes of the FIC intervention for residents with dementia and their family and staff caregivers were assessed in a study funded by the National Institute of Nursing Research (RO1-NRO1689). A quasi-experimental design with nonequivalent groups and repeated pretest and posttest measures was employed to examine the effects of the FIC intervention on family, staff, and resident outcomes. Fourteen nursing homes in Iowa and Wisconsin with designated SCUs for individuals with dementia were recruited for the study. The nursing homes were grouped into pairs matched on ownership type (private nonprofit, private for-profit, and public) and SCU size. One nursing home in each pair was randomly assigned to be an experimental site and the other to be a control site. All individuals with dementia who were residing in or admitted to the SCUs during a 2-year period and their family members were eligible to participate. The primary nurse or social worker in the SCU identified the family caregiver most closely involved with each resident's care and asked that family caregiver if he or she would be willing to be contacted to participate in the study. All staff assigned to work on the SCUs or who had a caseload assignment on the SCUs were eligible to participate. Assignment of staff was nonrandom and done by the agencies' administrations.

Two hundred family members were enrolled in the study (Maas, Swanson, et al., 2000). Of these enrollees, 185 were considered eligible and completed baseline questionnaires. Their average age was 61 years. The family member sample was predominantly Caucasian (94%), and about three fourths were women. Nearly 60% had more than a high school education. Forty percent were daughters, 14% sons, 21% wives, 7% husbands, 10% other relatives (niece, grandchild, sibling, and so forth), and 8% nonrelative friends or guardians. When grouped into those of the same generation as the resident and those of a younger generation, 33% were of the same generation (mean age = 73 years) and 67% were of a younger generation (mean age = 55 years). The

165 residents to whom the family caregiver participants were related had been in the nursing home a median duration of approximately $1^{1}/_{2}$ years (565 days), with a range of 23 days to 10.8 years. Fifty-seven of the residents had been in another nursing home previously for a median duration of 6 months, with a range of 30 days to 7 years.

A total of 845 staff members agreed to participate in the research. Of these, 93% were Caucasian and 92% were women. Their average age was 37 years, and the median length of employment in their current position was 5 years, with a range of 0 to 50 years. Forty-eight percent were nursing assistants, 5% were medication aides, 13% were registered nurses (RNs), 10% were licensed practical nurses (LPNs), and 10% were housekeeping, laundry, or maintenance personnel. Remaining staff (13%) classified themselves as activities technician/assistant/therapist, dietitian, social worker, administrator, ward or unit clerk, occupational therapy technician/assistant, physical therapy technician/assistant, speech-language therapist, music therapist, and religious activities director. The median number of months working at the facility for all staff was 24 months, with a range of 0 to 432 months.

Procedure

A 9-month trial of the FIC intervention was completed for each family member. Family member outcome measures were collected bimonthly, with a baseline and four follow-up assessments. Staff members were recruited to participate and, following consent, staff outcome measures were collected at baseline prior to the training sessions and every 6 months throughout the 2-year period of the study in each nursing home. The enrollment period and timing of follow-ups differed between family and staff participants for both practical and theoretical reasons. Practically, retention of family caregivers beyond 9 months was expected to be problematic, and staff data collection more frequently than every 6 months was not feasible for the participating institutions. Theoretically, the intervention was expected to be of more central significance for family caregivers than for staff members, and therefore the impact was expected to be more immediate for family members.

Once staff training was completed, family members were recruited to participate and informed consent was obtained from them. Implementation of the FIC intervention protocol began as soon as the first family members' baseline measures (pretest) were obtained. Interviews also were conducted with each family member at baseline and during months 5 and 9.

Outcome Measures

Family

Family members' outcomes were measured by the 81-item Family Perceptions of Caregiving Role (FPCR) instrument and the 51-item Family Perceptions of Care Tool (FPCT). The investigators developed these instruments and pretested them for reliability and validity (Maas & Buckwalter, 1990). Items in both are rated on a 7-point Likert scale. Directionality varies across items and is reconciled by rescoring items within a scale to achieve consistency. The FPCR contains four scales to measure four dimensions of role stress: *loss* of aspects of the relationship with the person with dementia, *guilt* from perceived failure in caregiving, *captivity* resulting from obligations of caregiving, and *conflict* with staff over caregiving. The FPCT contains four scales to measure perceived satisfaction with *physical care, activities* for residents, unit *management,* and staff *disregard* (lack of consideration) for the resident and family member. For this study, the scales of the family instruments were assembled into four clusters corresponding with the four aspects of the caregiving role described in the theoretical model. Table 8.1 shows the correspondence between the aspects of caregiving role, the character of the clusters for both types of caregivers, and the scales in each cluster. Cronbach's alpha (i.e., internal reliability) for each scale is also included in this table.

Staff

Staff completed the 78-item Staff Perceptions of Caregiving Role (SPCR) instrument, the 43-item Caregiver Stress Inventory (CSI), and the 16-item Attitudes Toward Families Checklist (AFC). All of the measures were developed by the investigators and were pretested for reliability and validity in earlier work (Maas & Buckwalter, 1990). All items on these instruments are rated on a 7-point Likert scale. The SPCR measures four dimensions of staff caregiving role stress. *Task burden* constitutes the costs of caregiving, such as feeling anger or feeling overworked. *Role inadequacy* is the feeling that there are no benefits from caregiving, in that what one does fails to help the residents with dementia. *Dominion* reflects the attitude that staff should be in control of caregiving. *Exclusion* is the disposition that family members should not participate in caregiving in the nursing home; exclusion is conceptually distinct from dominion because family members conceivably may participate extensively without being involved in decision making regarding care. The CSI measures four dimensions of stress related to resident *aggression, inappropriate behavior, safety* (potential for *harm to* residents), and *resources* available to staff to enhance care for people with dementia. The AFC measures staff perceptions of whether family caregivers are *disruptive,* whether they are *irrelevant* to care, and whether they should be *partners* in care. Cronbach's alphas for all of the staff outcome scales are presented in Table 8.7. The scales of the staff measures, like the scales of the family measures, were organized into four clusters corresponding with the four significant aspects of the caregiving role (see Table 8.7).

Residents

Resident characteristics were included in the analyses for family members as control variables. The 28-item Functional Abilities Checklist (FAC) was used to measure care recipients' characteristics related to dementia at baseline. The FAC has components measuring *disruptive behavior* (socially inappropriate and agitated/aggressive behavior) and *functional level* (cognitive and self-care abilities). Internal consistency reliability coefficients with the baseline data were .86 for disruptive behavior and .87 for functional level. Because toileting in particular appears related to the decision for nursing home admission (Newman, 2003), the Minimum Data Set toileting ability item also was used as a predictor.

Data Analysis

Because of space limitations and the purpose of the chapter, a complete explanation of the data analysis is not presented here but can be obtained in an article published by Maas et al. (2004). A hierarchical linear modeling (HLM) approach (Bryk & Raudenbush, 1992; Raudenbush, Bryk, & Congdon, 2001) was used to analyze the effects of the FIC intervention on the outcome measures over time. This approach was useful for this study because it does not require complete data

Table 8.7.   Intervention effects for family and staff with unadjusted p values and p values adjusted

	Family caregiver outcomes			
Measure	Estimated change by 9 months	9-month change/ baseline SD	Unadjusted p value	Adjusted p value
Emotional reaction to care recipient				
Guilt			.221	.351
Captivity	−.80	.20	.024	.041
Loss	−.68	.45	.001	.003
Relationship with staff				
Conflict			.417	.534
Disregard	−.72	.62	.001	.002
Perceptions of care				
Physical care	.58	.34	.010	.014
Activities	.47	.38	.001	.002
Perceptions of management				
Management			.965	.965

	Staff caregiver outcomes			
Measure	Estimated change by 18 months	18-month change/ baseline SD	Unadjusted p value	Adjusted p value
Emotional reaction to care recipient's				
Inappropriate behavior			.522	.808
Aggression	.17	.13	.003	.007
Perceived relationship with family				
Exclusion			.716	.940
Partnership			.665	.907
Disruption	−.14	.14	.007	.016
Dominion	−.24	.26	< .001	.002
Irrelevance	−.20		< .001	.002
Perceptions of caregiving				
Resident harm			.849	.985
Task burden			.284	.526
Role inadequacy			.277	.515
Perceived organizational support				
Resources			.99	.99

from participants in order for them to be included in the analysis. The final scheduled data collection was completed for 83 family members and 206 staff members. Some staff and family members missed interim data collections altogether, while completing later data collections.

RESULTS

Beneficial intervention effects were found in three of the four areas of family caregiver outcomes and one of the four areas of staff outcomes. In general, effect sizes were larger for family than staff caregiver outcomes, even when considering shorter time periods for family than for staff. No significant effects were found for residents with dementia. Table 8.7 presents intervention effects for family and staff outcomes.

Family Outcome Measures

Family Members' Emotional Reactions to Care Recipient

The measures of family caregiver emotional reactions were the loss, guilt, and captivity scales of the FPCR. The intervention and comparison groups did not differ significantly at baseline on any of the measures. The FIC intervention had significant effects on family members' feelings of loss and captivity. Loss scores increased significantly ($p < .01$) over time for the same-generation caregivers in the comparison group while remaining constant for the same-generation caregivers in the intervention group. Loss scores for younger generation caregivers, which were lower at baseline than those of the same-generation caregivers, remained constant over time in both the intervention and comparison groups. For captivity, scores decreased over time for those in the intervention group ($p < .05$), regardless of generation, whereas there was no change over time for the comparison group.

The relationship of other variables to loss and captivity scores was also investigated. It was found that baseline loss scores were higher when disruptive behavior by the resident was higher ($p < .001$). Captivity scores at baseline were higher for those in the same generation, higher as disruptive behavior was higher, and lower as the length of time in the facility increased ($p < .05$ for all).

Family Members' Perceptions of Relationships with Staff

Two family outcome measures reflect relationships with staff, the conflict scale of the FPCR and the disregard scale of the FPCT. The intervention and comparison groups did not differ on adjusted mean baseline scores for either of these measures. There was no intervention effect on family members' scores on conflict with staff. For the disregard scale, the same-generation comparison group has a significant increase ($p < .01$; i.e., scores become more negative concerning staff), whereas the same-generation intervention group shows no change over time. In both the younger generation comparison and intervention groups, no change over time was evident.

Family Members' Perceptions of Care

There were two measures of a family member's perceptions of the care provided to his or her relative in the SCU, the physical care scale and the activities scale. An intervention effect was found for both. Evaluations of physical care did not change over time for the comparison group, but increased significantly for the intervention group ($p < .01$). The intervention effect for the activities scale again differed by generation. The trend for the same-generation comparison group was significantly negative (adjusted $p = .001$) in comparison with the flat trend for the same-generation intervention group and the younger generation comparison and intervention groups.

Family Members' Perceptions of Management Effectiveness

No intervention effect on the management scale was found ($p = .84$). Baseline values were higher if the family caregiver could travel to the nursing home ($p < .001$), increased as the toileting ability of the resident decreased ($p < .01$), and decreased as the disruptive behavior of the resident increased ($p < .01$).

Staff Outcome Measures

Staff Emotional Reactions to Care Recipient

Two staff outcome scales measured staff stress from interaction with residents, the inappropriate behavior stress scale and the aggressive behavior stress scale. (Resident harm stress is considered a role performance measure, although it also concerns interactions with residents.)

Of the two measures, the aggressive behavior stress scale showed a statistically significant intervention effect. That effect was not beneficial. Comparison group staff scores did not change over time, whereas the intervention group reported significant increases ($p < .01$), although the rate of increase declined over time ($p < .01$).

For inappropriate behavior stress, the higher the education level of the job category, the more desirable the baseline score on all these measures ($p < .05$). The longer the time in the occupation, the higher (worse) the scores were ($p < .05$ for all), consistent with an expectation of burnout.

Staff Perceptions of Relationships with Family

Five staff outcome measures concern staff relationships with family caregivers or staff members' evaluation of the role of family caregivers. These are the dominion, exclusion, family irrelevance, disruption by family, and partnership scales.

Intervention and comparison groups did not differ on any of these measures at baseline. Three of the scales concerned with relationships show beneficial effects from the intervention: the dominion ($p < .01$; see Table 8.7), the disruption by family ($p < .05$), and the irrelevance of family ($p < .01$) scales. Scores on all three scales declined over time for intervention group staff, whereas the scores for the comparison group did not change.

In investigations of the effects of other variables, job classification was found to have a significant effect on the baseline value for all of these scales. In general, staff with a higher education level rated family caregivers more favorably ($p < .05$ for all). That is, RNs had more desirable scores than LPNs and similarly educated staff, who in turn had more desirable scores than certified nursing assistants and similarly educated staff. For both disruption ($p < .001$) and dominion ($p < .05$), the longer the staff member had been in the occupation, the *less* favorable toward families was the score. For both dominion ($p < .05$) and exclusion scores ($p < .01$), men tended to have higher (less favorable to families) scores than women.

Staff Reactions to Care Role

Three staff outcome measures reflected staff reactions to their role in providing care to residents, the role inadequacy scale, the task burden, and the resident harm stress scale. No intervention effects were found for any of these three measures. In general, the higher the education level of the staff member, the more desirable the baseline score on the measure, except that RNs experienced more resident harm stress than other staff, probably reflecting their greater sense of responsibility.

Staff Perceptions of Organizational Support

One scale, the resource deficiency stress scale, assessed staff perceptions of support from the organization for carrying out their caregiving responsibilities. No intervention effect was found for this measure ($p = .99$).

DISCUSSION

Baseline interviews with family members in the FIC study revealed that the transition to the nursing home is a particularly difficult time for family members (Butcher et al., 2001; Hagen, 2001). Relationships with residents following relocation are difficult for family caregivers, exacerbate feelings of guilt and loss, and produce uncertainty about how to perform their changing roles. The study results indicate that implementing the FIC intervention in nursing home SCUs ameliorates feelings of loss and captivity, increases satisfaction with physical care, and prevents deterioration of satisfaction with the activities of residents over time for family caregivers who are of the same generation as the care recipient, most of whom are spouses. Perceived relationships of the family caregivers with staff members and residents also became more favorable after implementation of the intervention, which produced more positive staff perceptions of their relationships with family members—less inclination to control and to view family members as disruptive and irrelevant to the care of residents. These results support other research findings indicating that, in family-oriented nursing homes, trust in the staff was reported and mutual affection in relationships was apparent (Duncan & Morgan, 1994; Friedemann et al., 1997).

The positive effects of the FIC with older, mostly spouse-caregivers as opposed to younger caregivers may have occurred because spouses feel the loss of their mates more acutely than do the children of parents with dementia and are also more apt to feel trapped by obligations to care for their mates. For same-generation family members, the loss and captivity may be felt even more as the disease manifests in behaviors that make relating difficult. Over time, older family caregivers may find ways to feel less obliged as they adjust to care provided in the

SCU, yet feel responsible when there is more risk for or actual instance of adverse occurrences, such as the resident falling. Younger family members may have more competing role expectations than older members, causing them to be more detached in their caregiving and less influenced by the FIC intervention.

Although the findings support the conclusion that the FIC intervention had important beneficial effects on both family and staff caregivers, the effects fell short of reflecting full partnerships between family and staff caregivers, and there were fewer positive effects for younger generation family members, mostly children of the residents with dementia. The intervention did not influence the perceived conflict with staff on the part of family caregivers or the perception of a partnership with family caregivers on the part of staff. Furthermore, the effects of the intervention did not include a significant reduction in staff stress associated with caregiving task burden or role inadequacy. Stress associated with the aggressive behaviors of residents increased initially, with some tempering as the study trial progressed.

Implementing nursing interventions in nursing home settings is very difficult because of a number of constraints, such as staff turnover, understaffing, institutional routines, and a lack of RN leadership (Maas, Kelley, Park, & Specht, 2002). Before any of the quantitative results of the study were known, the master's-level nurse clinicians responsible for implementing the intervention anticipated that the impact of the intervention on staff might be limited because the clinicians felt the nursing home administrators and the nursing home staff never really adopted the intervention as their own. Rather, it seemed that staff members saw it as something they did for the research team. Positive results were achieved, but even better results might be achieved if the commitment of the nursing staff to the intervention were stronger. Finding ways to achieve greater staff ownership and compliance with the intervention may increase its positive effects on both family and staff members.

One way to improve staff commitment that is suggested by these results is to encourage RNs to participate and provide greater leadership to unlicensed assisting personnel. Not surprisingly, RNs had the most family-friendly scores of all occupational groups on all family-related measures, suggesting that RNs could be leaders in promoting family involvement with unlicensed assisting personnel, who make up the bulk of the nursing staff and who have the most direct contacts with residents and families (Duncan & Morgan, 1994).

Clearly, different interventions need to be designed and the FIC protocol needs to be adjusted and tested to improve outcomes for

younger generation family members and staff, or both. Adjustment of
the FIC intervention and assessment of factors influencing its effectiveness should target specific family members (e.g., same generation versus
not same generation; spouse, child, sibling, niece/nephew). Mutual
goals for residents and the type and extent of involvement may need
to be more carefully designed for each type of family caregiver. "Dosage"
(extent of family involvement) of the FIC intervention may influence
effectiveness. Dosage was documented during the FIC study, but an
analysis of the effects of dosage on outcomes has not been completed
and reported. Future research should also incorporate systemwide strategies to achieve greater integration of interventions with setting culture
and administration.

The research staff also noted that family members, although desir-
ing to participate more in the resident's care, often had few ideas
about what they could do. As the resident's stay in the nursing home
continued, family members often became more uncertain and lacking
in information about the resident's day-to-day abilities and behavior.
Staff members typically did not actively help family members remain
optimally informed or explore various ways that they could be more
involved. This may be one reason why the intervention had fewer
positive effects for younger generation family caregivers. The intervention included education for all staff members in the intervention sites
on the rationale for FIC and how to develop a partnership agreement,
including role playing and case examples of family participation in care.
The advantages of family involvement in assisting staff with their care
activities and in providing helpful information about the resident were
emphasized. Special sessions were also held with the RN or social
worker on each SCU who would take the lead in negotiating the partnership agreements with family members. Too often, however, the
leadership expected was lacking because of turnover and the limited
engagement of an RN with nursing assistants in providing resident care.

Implementation of the FIC intervention as soon as, or even before,
the resident with dementia is admitted to the nursing home may be
especially important for family members. Because nearly all of the
family members participating in this study had relatives who had been
residing in the nursing home for at least 6 months, it was not possible
to determine whether there were differential effects for family members
with newly admitted relatives and those with relatives who were long-
term residents. However, analysis of the interviews provided an in-
depth view of the perspective of family members and indicated that
they often had concerns about care but were reluctant to express those

concerns to staff members. This finding implies that the intervention might be more effective if it were implemented with the staff assuming a more inclusive and less governing role with family members and before family members established a pattern of deference to staff members in decision making.

If nursing homes wish to realize the benefits of increasing family involvement through the FIC intervention, leadership demonstrating full and active commitment to implementing the intervention is essential. It is important that long-term care facility leaders and policy makers define family–staff partnerships as desirable and that the support needed for staff members to implement the intervention is provided Although further research is needed to test the effects of the FIC on family, staff, and resident outcomes, the results of the current study suggest that it has much potential. It seems probable that staff members who learn to work with families as partners *and* as clients will experience greater role adequacy and job satisfaction through the achievement of more positive outcomes for families and residents. The positive results of the FIC intervention in nursing home SCUs as reported in other studies (Bauer & Nay, 2003; Keefe & Fancey, 2000) also suggest that the intervention should be useful for family and staff caregivers of other nursing home populations and for residents in other settings.

With the increasing number of individuals with dementia and with fewer family members able to devote themselves to full-time caregiving, the number of people with dementia in nursing homes and other long-term care facilities will continue to increase. Thus, it will be important for family and staff caregivers to develop satisfying roles in long-term care facilities, roles that minimize the stress of continued caregiving. Implications for nursing education, practice, and research and for health policy are apparent. Further use and testing of the FIC or similar interventions in nursing homes is important and requires a more sustained research focus in the future. Nursing education programs need to emphasize leadership and partnering with families in caregiving. Finally, greater efforts are needed to revise health policies so that shared caregiving with families led by sufficient numbers of RNs and assisting staff is a standard that is adequately funded.

CONCLUSION

Since completing the FIC study, the authors of this chapter are unaware of any nursing home setting in which the intervention has been formally adopted. They have observed some change, however, in the way some nursing homes work with families; that is, family members are included more in decisions, are asked to share more information with staff, and are helped to find ways to make their interactions with residents more meaningful and satisfying. Since the FIC Evidence-Based Protocol was published (Kelley, Specht, & Maas, 2000), the authors have received numerous requests for more information, use of measures, and collaboration. The authors' sense is that the principles of FIC are disseminating slowly and prompting greater awareness of the need for and benefits of family–staff partnerships. Nurses, however, are often reluctant to formalize a family–staff agreement. Most view the agreement as asking the family to help them, rather than seeing it as a collaboration (with the resident when possible) in how to meet the resident's needs, identifying what the family can and will do, and how the staff will support family efforts. The authors also continue to observe daily how long-term care policies that are based on a medical–custodial paradigm discourage the use of the FIC and other actions to improve the quality of care and life of older adults and their families. Combined with the bureaucracy of institutions and chronic under-staffing of nurse leaders with gerontological training, it is understand-able why interventions such as FIC often are not implemented. Clearly, much more work is needed that focuses on translating the FIC interven-tion into practice and on influencing changes in long-term care policies that impede the use of evidence-based best nursing practices.

Based on our experience with the research and our observations of the research sites and other nursing homes, we have noted several key actions for successfully implementing the FIC intervention:

1. RNs must believe in the need for the intervention and provide leadership for assisting staff members in implementing the partner-ship protocol.

2. Agency administration must be committed to the intervention and support its implementation.

3. Assisting staff members must be actively involved in each step of implementing and evaluating the intervention.

4. The FIC intervention should be incorporated with quarterly confer-ences that are held with the resident and family.

5. Policies and environmental factors that discourage or prevent implementation of the FIC intervention (e.g., supplies; privacy for

family and resident interactions; prohibitions on family members performing physical care activities such as bathing, ambulating, and toileting) should be reviewed by administration and eliminated.

6. A consistent person should be identified for family members to contact with questions, concerns, and recommendations.

7. The interventions should be implemented with families whom the staff has identified as most difficult. Dramatic changes in the relationships often result, making it easy for staff members to see the advantages of FIC.

REFERENCES

Acton, G.J., & Kang, J. (2001). Interventions to reduce the burden of caregiving for an adult with dementia: A meta-analysis. *Research in Nursing & Health, 24*, 349–360.

Bauer, M., & Nay, R. (2003). Family and staff partnerships in long-term care. *Journal of Gerontological Nursing, 29*(10), 46–53.

Bonder, B.R. (1986). Family systems and Alzheimer's disease: An approach to treatment. *Physical and Occupational Therapy in Geriatrics, 5*(2), 13–24.

Bowers, B.J. (1988). Family perceptions of care in a nursing home. *The Gerontologist, 28*(3), 361–368.

Bryk, A.S., & Raudenbush, S.W. (1992). *Hierarchical linear models.* Newbury Park, CA: Sage.

Butcher, H.K., Holkup, P.A., Park, M., & Maas, M. (2001). Thematic analysis of the experience of making a decision to place a family member with Alzheimer's disease in a special care unit. *Research in Nursing & Health, 24*, 470–480.

Canadian Study of Health and Aging Working Group. (2002). Patterns and health effects of caring for people with dementia: The impact of changing cognitive and residential status. *The Gerontologist, 42*, 643–652.

Chang, B.L. (1999). Cognitive-behavioural intervention for homebound caregivers of persons with dementia. *Nursing Research, 48*, 173–182.

Connell, C.M., Janevic, M.R., & Gallant, M.P. (2001). The costs of caring: Impact of dementia on family caregivers. *Journal of Geriatric Psychiatry and Neurology, 14*, 179–187.

Dellasega, C., & Mastrian, K. (1995). The process and consequences of institutionalizing an elder. *Western Journal of Nursing Research, 17*, 123–140.

Duncan, M.T., & Morgan, D.L. (1994). Sharing the caring: Family caregivers' views of their relationships with nursing home staff. *The Gerontologist, 34*, 235–244.

Fink, S., & Picot, S. (1995). Nursing home placement decisions and post placement experiences of African American and European American caregivers. *Journal of Gerontological Nursing, 21*(12), 35–42.

Friedemann, M., Montgomery, R.J., Maiberger, B., & Smith, A.A. (1997). Family involvement in the nursing home: Family-oriented practices and staff–family relationships. *Research in Nursing & Health, 20,* 527–537.

Friedemann, M., Montgomery, R., Rice, C., & Farrell, L. (1999). Family involvement in the nursing home. *Western Journal of Nursing Research, 21,* 549–567.

Gaugler, J.E., Anderson, K.A., Zarit, S.H., & Pearlin, L.I. (2004). Family involvement in nursing homes: Effects on stress and well-being. *Aging and Mental Health, 8,* 65–75.

Gaugler, J.E., Pearlin, L.I., Leitsch, S.A., & Davey, A. (2001). Relinquishing in-home dementia care: Difficulties and perceived helpfulness during the nursing home transition. *American Journal of Alzheimer's Disease & Other Dementias, 16,* 32–42.

Gaugler, J.E., Zarit, S.H., & Pearlin, L.I. (2003). Family involvement following institutionalization: Modeling nursing home visits over time. *International Journal of Aging and Human Development, 57,* 91–117.

Goode, K., Haley, W., Roth, D., & Ford, G. (1998). Predicting longitudinal changes in caregiver physical and mental health: A stress process model. *Health Psychology, 17,* 190–198.

Grant, I., Adler, K., Patterson, T., Dimsdale, J., Ziegler, M., & Irwing, M. (2002). Health consequences of Alzheimer's caregiving transitions: Effects of placement and bereavement. *Psychosomatic Medicine, 64,* 477–486.

Hagen, B. (2001). Nursing home placement: Factors affecting caregivers' decisions to place family members with dementia. *Journal of Gerontological Nursing, 27*(2), 44–53.

Hall, G.R., & Buckwalter, K.C. (1987). Progressively lowered stress threshold: A conceptual model for care of adults with Alzheimer's disease. *Archives of Psychiatric Nursing, 1,* 399–406.

Hardy, M.E., & Conway, M. (1978). *Role therapy: Perspectives for health professionals.* New York: Appleton-Century-Crofts.

Jablonski, R.A.S., Reed, D., & Maas, M. (2005). Effect of family involvement in core intervention on cognitive functional outcomes of institutionalized elders with Alzheimer's disease and related dementias. *Journal of Gerontological Nursing, 3*(16), 38–48.

Kahana, E. (1982). A congruence model of person–environment interaction. In P. Lawton, P. Windley, & T. Byerts (Eds.), *Aging and the environment: Theoretical approaches* (pp. 97–121). New York: Springer.

Keefe, J., & Fancey, P. (2000). The care continues: Responsibility for elderly relatives before and after admission to a long term care facility. *Family Relations, 49,* 235–244.

Kelley, L.S., Specht, J.K., & Maas, M.L. (2000). Family involvement in care: A research-based protocol for persons with dementia or other chronic illnesses. *Journal of Gerontological Nursing, 26*(2), 13–21.

Kelley, L., Swanson, E., Maas, M., & Tripp-Reimer, T. (1999). Family visitation on special care units. *Journal of Gerontological Nursing, 25*(2), 14–21.

Kellett, U.M. (1998). Meaning-making for family carers in nursing homes. *International Journal of Nursing Practice, 4*(2), 113–119.

Lawton, M.P. (1982). Competence, environmental press and the adaptation of older people. In M.P. Lawton, P. Windley, & T. Byerts (Eds.), *Aging and the environment: Theoretical approaches* (pp. 33–59). New York: Springer.

Maas, M., & Buckwalter, K. (1990). *Final report: Phase II Nursing Evaluation Research: Alzheimer's Care Unit* (Research Grant, National Institute of Nursing Research RO1-NRO1689). Rockville, MD: National Institutes of Health.

Maas, M., Buckwalter, K., Swanson, E., & Mobily, P. (1994). Training key to job satisfaction. *Journal of Long Term Care Administration, 22*(1), 23–26.

Maas, M., Buckwalter, K., Swanson, E., Specht, J., Hardy, M., & Tripp-Reimer, T. (1994). The caring partnership: Staff and families of persons institutionalized with Alzheimer's disease. *Journal of Alzheimer's Disease and Related Disorders, 9*, 21–30.

Maas, M., Kelley, L., Park, M., & Specht, J.P. (2002). Issues in conducting research in nursing homes. *Western Journal of Nursing Research, 24*, 373–389.

Maas, M., Reed, D., Park, M., Specht, J., Schutte, D., Kelley, L., et al. (2004). Outcomes of family involvement in care intervention for caregivers of individuals with dementia. *Nursing Research, 53*, 76–86.

Maas, M., Reed, D., Specht, J., Swanson, S., Tripp-Reimer, T., Buckwalter, K., et al. (1992). Family involvement in care: Negotiated family–staff partnerships in special care units for persons with dementia. In S.G. Funk, E.M. Tomquist, M.T. Champagne, & R.A. Wiese (Eds.), *Key aspects of elder care: Managing falls, incontinence, and cognitive impairment* (pp. 330–345). New York: Springer.

Maas, M., & Swanson, E. (1992). *Nursing interventions for Alzheimer's: Family role trials* (Research Grant, National Institute of Nursing Research RO1-NRO1689). Rockville, MD: National Institutes of Health.

Maas, M., Swanson, E., Buckwalter, K., Specht, J., Tripp-Reimer, T., Lenth, R., et al. (2000). *Final Report: Nursing interventions for Alzheimer's: Family role trials* (Research Grant, National Institute of Nursing Research RO1-NRO1689). Rockville, MD: National Institutes of Health.

Magaziner, J., German, P., Zimmerman, S.I., Hebel, J.R., Burton, L., Gruber-Baldini, A.L., et al. (2000). The prevalence of dementia in a statewide sample of new nursing home admissions aged 65 and older: Diagnosis by expert panel. *The Gerontologist, 40*, 663–672.

Montgomery, R.J. (1982). The impact of institutional care policies on family integration. *The Gerontologist, 22*, 54–58.

Montgomery, R.J., & Montoro, J. (1995, November). *Family members as the "other clients" in the nursing home setting.* Paper presented at the 48th annual Scientific Meeting of the Gerontological Society of America, Los Angeles.

Moss, M.S., Lawton, M.P., Kleban, M.H., & Duhamel, L. (1993). Time use of caregivers of impaired elders before and after institutionalization. *Journal of Gerontology, 48*(3), S102–S111.

O'Neill, G., & Ross, M.M. (1991). Burden of care: An important concept for nurses. *Health Care for Women International, 12*, 111–122.

Ostwald, S.K., Hepburn, K.W., Caron, W., Burns, T., & Mantell, R. (1999). Reducing caregiver burden: A randomized psychoeducational intervention for caregivers of persons with dementia. *The Gerontologist, 39*, 299–309.

Parr, J. (1980). The interaction of persons and living arrangements. In L.W. Poon (Ed)., *Aging in the 1980s: Psychological issues* (pp. 397–407). Washington, DC: American Psychological Association.

Pinquart, M., & Sorensen, S. (2003a). Associations of stressors and uplifts of caregiving with caregiver burden and depressive mood: A meta-analysis.

Journals of Gerontology. Series B, Psychological Sciences and Social Sciences, 58, P112–P128.

Pinquart, M., & Sorensen, S. (2003b). Differences between caregivers and noncaregivers in psychological health and physical health: A meta-analysis. *Psychology and Aging, 18,* 250–267.

Raudenbush, S., Bryk, A., & Congdon, R. (2001). HLM, Version 5.04 [Computer software]. Chicago: Scientific Software International.

Rubin, A., & Shuttlesworth, G.E. (1983). Engaging families as support resources in nursing home care: Ambiguity in the subdivision of tasks. *The Gerontologist, 23,* 632–636.

Ryan, A.A., & Scullion, H.F. (2000). Family and staff perceptions of the role of families in nursing homes. *Journal of Advanced Nursing, 32,* 626–634.

Specht, J.P., Kelley, L.S., Manion, P., Maas, M.L., Reed, D., & Rantz, M. (2000). Who's the boss? Family/staff partnership in care of persons with dementia. *Nursing Administration Quarterly, 24*(3), 64–77.

Spencer, B. (1991). The role of families in dementia care units. In D.H. Coons (Ed.), *Specialized dementia care units* (pp. 189–204). Baltimore: Johns Hopkins University Press.

Tornatore, J., & Grant, L. (2002). Burden among family caregivers of persons with Alzheimer's disease in nursing homes. *The Gerontologist, 42,* 497–506.

Travis, S.S. (1996). Formal long-term care networks: Forming a partnership with gerontological nurses. *Journal of Gerontological Nursing, 22*(12), 21–24.

Unverzagt, F.W., Gao, S., Baiyewu, O., Ogunniyi, A.O., Gureje, O., Perkins, A., et al. (2001). Prevalence of cognitive impairment: Data from the Indianapolis Study of Health and Aging. *Neurology, 57,* 1655–1662.

Vitaliano, P.P., Zhang, J., & Scanlan, J.M. (2003). Is caregiving hazardous to one's physical health? A meta-analysis. *Psychological Bulletin, 129,* 946–972.

Volicer, L., McKee, A., & Hewitt, S. (2001). Dementia. *Neurologic Clinics, 19,* 867–885.

Wilcox, S., & King, A. (1999). Sleep complaints in older women who are family caregivers. *Journals of Gerontology. Series B, Psychological Sciences and Social Sciences, 54,* 189–198.

Wilkens, D.S., Castle, S., Heck, E., Tanzy, K., & Fahey, J. (1999). Immune function, mood and perceived burden among caregivers participating in a psychoeducational intervention. *Psychiatric Services, 50,* 747–749.

Wright, L.K., Clipp, E.C., & George, L.K. (1993). Health consequences of caregiver stress. *Medicine, Exercise, Nutrition, and Health, 2*(4), 181–195.

RESOURCES

The Family Involvement in Care study was funded by the National Institute of Nursing Research (RO1-NRO1689; Meridean L. Maas, Principal Investigator). For additional information, please contact

Janet K. Pringle Specht, Ph.D., RN
432 Nursing Building

50 Newton Road
The University of Iowa
College of Nursing
Iowa City, IA 52242
E-mail: Janet-specht@uiowa.edu
Telephone: 319-335-6518

David Reed, Ph.D.
414 Nursing Building
50 Newton Road
The University of Iowa
College of Nursing
Iowa City, IA 52242
E-mail: david-reed@uiowa.edu
Telephone: 319-335-7078

Meridean L. Maas, Ph.D., RN
430 Nursing Building
50 Newton Road
The University of Iowa
College of Nursing
Iowa City, IA 52242
E-mail: Meridean-maas@uiowa.edu
Telephone: 319-335-7107

Additional Resources

Alzheimer's Association. (1995). *Activity programming for persons with dementia: A source book.* Chicago: Author.

Basting, A.D., & Kellick, J. (2003). *The arts and dementia care: A resource guide.* Brooklyn, NY: The National Center for Creative Aging.

Bell, V., Troxel, D., Cox, T., & Hamon, R. (2004). *The best friends book of Alzheimer's activities.* Baltimore: Health Professions Press.

Gerdner, L. (1998). *Research-based protocol: Individualized music.* Iowa City: The University of Iowa Gerontological Nursing Interventions Research Center, Research Development and Dissemination Core.

Harvath, T.A., Archbold, P.G., Stewart, B.J., Gadow, S., Kirschling, J.M., Miller, L., et al. (1994). Establishing partnerships with family caregivers: Local and cosmopolitan knowledge. *Journal of Gerontological Nursing, 22*(2), 29–35.

Iowa Intervention Project. (2000). *Nursing interventions classification (NIC)* (J. McCloskey & G. Bulechek, Eds.). St. Louis: Mosby.

Iowa Outcomes Project. (2000). *Classification of nursing outcomes (NOC)* (M. Johnson & M. Maas, Eds.). St. Louis: Mosby.

Kelley, L.S., Specht, J.P., & Maas, M.L. (1999). *Research based protocol: Family Involvement in Care for Persons with Dementia (FIC)*. Iowa City: The University of Iowa Gerontological Nursing Interventions Research Center, Research Development and Dissemination Core.

Logue, R.M. (2003). Maintaining family connectedness in long-term care: An advanced practice approach to family-centered nursing homes. *Journal of Gerontological Nursing, 29*(6), 24–31.

Schulz, R., Belle, S.H., Czaja, S.J., McGinnis, K.A., Stevens, A., & Zhang, S. (2004). Long-term care placement of dementia patients and caregiver health and well-being. *JAMA, 292,* 961–967.

8

Appendix

Family and Staff Partnership Agreement
Staff Training Objectives for the FIC Intervention

Family and Staff
Partnership Agreement

Staff and family have agreed that they are partners in planning, providing, and evaluating care for _____ (Resident)

Family member(s) will do the following activities
(Please include frequency and amount of time for each activity):

_____

_____

_____

Staff will do the following activities
(Please include frequency and amount of time for each activity):

_____

_____

_____

Comments and explanations:

_____

_____

_____

Family member(s) signature(s) _____

Date _____

Facility staff signatures _____

Date _____

Research supported by NIH NINR funded grant, Nursing Interventions for Alzheimer's Family Role Trials, R01NR01869.

Staff Training Objectives for the FIC Intervention

SESSION 1: OVERVIEW OF CARE OF RESIDENTS WITH DEMENTIA AND THE ROLE OF FAMILY CAREGIVERS

At the completion of the presentation, the participant will be able to

1. Give an overview of dementia, including definition, stages, and common behavior problems

2. Describe principles of caring for residents with dementia

3. Demonstrate an understanding of the role transition of family members when their relatives are admitted to a nursing home

4. List common sources of family stress when considering admission of a relative to a nursing home

5. List common emotional reactions of family members during relocation of their relative to a nursing home

6. Discuss principles of interacting with family members of residents with dementia

SESSION 2: FAMILY INVOLVEMENT IN CARE (FIC) INTERVENTION

At the completion of this session, the participant will be able to

1. Describe the rationale and purpose of the family–staff partnership in the care of residents with dementia

2. Discuss the benefits of the family–staff partnership

3. Demonstrate familiarity with how the family–staff partnership and agreement are negotiated, evaluated, and renegotiated

4. List the four steps of the FIC intervention

5. Demonstrate familiarity with the FIC intervention procedures and forms

Promoting Family Involvement in Long-Term Care Settings:
A Guide to Programs that Work, edited by Joseph E. Gaugler
© Copyright 2005 by Health Professions Press, Inc. All rights reserved.

SESSION 3: FAMILY–STAFF PARTNERSHIP NEGOTIATION

At the completion of the session, participants will be able to

1. Describe the concept of role negotiation and the principles of the role negotiation process

2. Describe the concepts of conflict and conflict resolution

3. List examples of role conflict and family–staff conflict

4. Discuss how strategies for resolution of conflict are related to and inherent in the process of developing and implementing a family–staff agreement

5. Demonstrate role negotiation and the development of a family–staff agreement

6. Negotiate a family–staff agreement

9

Partners in Caregiving

Cooperative Communication Between Families and Nursing Homes

JULIE ROBISON AND KARL A. PILLEMER

Research has clearly demonstrated that family caregivers maintain close ties to relatives living in nursing homes (Duncan & Morgan, 1994; Tobin, 1995). However, many family members experience considerable stress regarding admission of their relative and developing relationships with the nursing home staff over long periods of time (Bauer & Nay, 2003; Hertzberg & Ekman, 1996; Tobin, 1995). Nursing home staff members report experiencing stress from multiple aspects of their jobs, including the pressure to work successfully with residents' families (Cohen-Mansfield, 1995; Heiselman & Noelker, 1991; Pillemer, Hegeman, Albright, & Henderson, 1998).

Litwak (1985) proposed a theoretical framework that may explain the difficulties staff and families experience in working together to provide care for residents. Basic differences between formal organizations, such as long-term care facilities, and families lead to a mismatch between the organization's structure and the resident care tasks performed. Organizations must adhere to formal rules, a bureaucratic structure, and impersonal relationships. Yet in nursing homes, many responsibilities call for personal care and attention to individual needs, tasks that may be more ideally suited for family members based on their attachment and long-term relationships to residents (Litwak, 1985; Litwak, Jessop, & Moulton, 1994, Pillemer et al., 2003).

The most common obstacles to good staff–family relationships fit into Litwak's (1985) theoretical framework (Logue, 2003). Staff and family members report different interpretations of which tasks each group should perform and how they should do them (Nolan & Dellasega, 1999; Stephens, Ogrocki, & Kinney, 1991). Staff uniformly report not having enough time to provide the care they would like to give to residents or to talk at any length with family members (Pillemer, 1996), and family members may be fearful about offering suggestions or complaining because of concerns that such comments might negatively affect the care staff members provide to the resident (Hertzberg & Ekman, 1996). These obstacles are compounded by significant cultural differences between staff members and residents and their families. For example, in some nursing homes (particularly in urban areas), a disproportionately minority staff cares for a predominantly white group of residents; similarly, differences in socioeconomic class often exist between residents and staff. Negative stereotypes held by both staff and families create another barrier (Specht et al., 2000). Some families perceive the staff as untrustworthy (Krause, Grant, & Long, 1999; Tobin, 1995) and feel they need to monitor staff behavior (Duncan & Morgan, 1994; Stull, Cosbey, Bowman, & McNutt, 1997), and staff members sometimes think families have unrealistic expectations of nursing home care (George & Maddox, 1989; Heiselman & Noelker, 1991).

Some research suggests that family involvement has positive benefits for residents and may even improve the family members' well-being as well (e.g., Gaugler, Anderson, Zarit, & Pearlin, 2004; Greene & Monahan, 1982; Noelker & Harel, 1978; Penrod, Kane, & Kane, 2000; Tornatore & Grant, 2004). Forging partnerships between staff members and families has the potential to further improve resident, staff, and family member quality of life. However, few programs exist that promote such cooperation and communication (Davis & Buckwalter, 2001; see Peak, 2000, for an example). Historically, programs have focused exclusively on family members, ignoring staff needs in developing successful relationships with families and neglecting to address issues at the administrative level.

Over the past 10 years, researchers from the Cornell Institute for Translational Research on Aging (CITRA), the Foundation for Long Term Care, and the Center on Aging at the University of Connecticut Health Center have developed two programs designed to remedy this situation. The first is a program to promote family and staff cooperation, known as Partners in Caregiving (PIC; Pillemer et al., 1998), with an adapted version for dementia units, Partners in Caregiving in the Special Care Unit (PIC-SCU) Environment. The second is a program focused on communication processes aimed at improving end-of-life care, called the Caring Communication program.

In particular, residents, family members, and staff members from dementia special care units (SCUs) stand to benefit from such programs. Residents with cognitive impairments are frequently unable to talk about their experiences in the facility or their past histories and preferences. Families are dependent on the staff for descriptions of life in the nursing home, and staff members can learn invaluable information about residents from their families. Unfortunately, interviews with both staff and family members indicate that sharing detailed information about residents is often inadequate and that families frequently feel there is no one with whom they can discuss this issue (Ekman & Norberg, 1988; Safford, 1989). Care practices that do not take into account residents' individual abilities, preferences, or dislikes can lead to undesirable behaviors. Communication of family members' knowledge about a resident's premorbid personality, as well as his or her disease history, to nursing home staff is critical for developing appropriate individualized care plans. Such communication may serve to increase understanding of, and perhaps reduce the expression of, behavioral symptoms in the nursing home.

CONCEPTUAL UNDERPINNINGS OF THE PARTNERS IN CAREGIVING PROGRAM

The PIC program consists of 1) parallel training sessions to enhance communication techniques and develop conflict-resolution skills with families and staff members, and 2) a subsequent meeting with families, staff members, and nursing home administrators to foster administrative support of the project's goals. This design draws on two mechanisms to effect changes in family and staff perceptions and behaviors. The first addresses the need to improve communication skills for both staff and family members. Research has demonstrated that training health professionals in cooperative communication is effective (Caris-Vehallen, Kerkstra, & Bensing, 1997; Greenberg, Doblin, Shapiro, Linn, & Wenger, 1993; Levinson & Roter, 1993; McCormick, Inui, & Roter, 1996). Evidence also exists that communication training can improve relations between families and community institutions such as schools (Cochran & Dean, 1991; Henderson & Berla, 1994). This latter research is particularly compelling as a model for addressing the institution–family disconnect in nursing homes described by Litwak (1985).

The second component of the program focuses on discussing and recommending changes in facility policies and procedures in the context of a joint meeting between families and facility staff members and administrators. Modeled on a successful program addressing relations between parents and teachers (Cochran & Dean, 1991), these sessions increase the sense of involvement and control for participants and create solidarity between staff and family members. Furthermore, they provide an opportunity for members of both groups to work toward consensus on changes in facility practices or policies with administrative support.

PROGRAM HISTORY AND EVALUATION OF THE PARTNERS IN CAREGIVING PROGRAM

Dr. Karl Pillemer from CITRA conducted pilot research when designing the PIC intervention. First, a survey of 218 New York nursing homes revealed persistent themes of distrust and misunderstanding between staff and family members. Nearly all participants expressed a need for improved communication between these groups. Second, Dr. Pillemer (in collaboration with the Foundation for Long Term Care, Albany, New York) designed and pilot-tested PIC. Results provided evidence of the program's effectiveness in improving communication and positive attitudes between nursing home staff and families, in addition to generating extremely high satisfaction ratings. Subsequently, the National Institute on Aging funded Dr. Pillemer to conduct a 5-year controlled-intervention study of PIC in units of 20 not-for-profit facilities in New York State. SCUs were deliberately excluded from the study because of the unique nature of family–staff interactions in these environments.

The controlled-intervention evaluation of PIC expanded upon prior efforts in five ways (Pillemer et al., 2003). First, the study design was based on a clearly articulated conceptual framework derived from both theory and empirical research on interpersonal interactions in long-term care settings. Second, the study was conducted in 20 skilled nursing facilities, allowing examination of the program's effectiveness across a range of settings. Third, rather than training only one of the two groups, both family and staff members from the same unit participated in the PIC workshops. Fourth, the program provided an opportunity for families and the staff to meet off the unit with facility administrators and to brainstorm about changes that would facilitate better family–staff relationships. Finally, the study assessed outcomes for both staff and family members.

The effects of the PIC program were evaluated via telephone interviews with family and staff members in the 20 participating facilities (Pillemer et al., 2003). Random assignment to the control or intervention group followed random selection of the 20 facilities from member facilities of the New York Association of Homes and Services for the Aging, the state's not-for-profit nursing home organization, in nine counties. Project staff randomly selected one unit in each of the 10 control facilities and two units in each of the 10 intervention facilities. Each intervention facility had an intervention unit that completed the PIC workshops, as well as a control unit. Randomization of the facilities was stratified by size and metropolitan/nonmetropolitan designation.

Telephone interviews were attempted with all nursing staff—registered nurses (RNs), licensed practical nurses (LPNs), and certified nursing assistants (CNAs)—on each unit (control and intervention) and with the designated responsible family member for each resident on the unit. For the intervention units, interviews occurred just prior to the PIC workshops and again 2 months and 6 months following the workshops. Control interviews followed the same time frame, with no intervening workshops. In the treatment units, 41% of family members participated in the training workshops and 82% of the staff participated. The family member participation rate reflects the decision to invite all responsible family members, many of who do not live near the facility or do not visit often. The unit-based, dual-group training design of the program makes it likely that even those who do not attend the workshops may notice an impact of the program through their interactions with staff and family members who did participate. Therefore, interviews were not limited to workshop attendees. Overall, 77% ($n = 932$) of family members and 80% ($n = 655$) of staff members completed baseline interviews. Attrition rates over the 6-month follow-up period ranged from 13% to 19%.

The program evaluation drew on data from the two follow-up assessments and on effects averaged over those two assessments (Pillemer et al., 2003). Because the program is of short duration and moderate intensity, effects might be expected to be strongest at the first follow-up, nearest to the time of intervention. The examination of the second follow-up gives an indication of the extent to which effects are sustained over a longer period of time. It is also possible that certain effects may take a longer time after involvement with the program to be manifested and would be apparent at the second follow-up. The test of effects averaged over the two follow-up assessments provides the best evidence of beneficial consequences of the program that are sustained over time and is the most powerful test of those effects.

Specific outcomes were measured at each time point for families and staff. Statistical analyses as well as measurement tools are described in detail elsewhere (Pillemer et al., 2003). Families' outcomes included their reports of conflict with staff, their attitudes about staff behaviors and staff empathy toward them, feelings of caregiver burden, and symptoms of depression. Staff members' outcomes included their perceptions of family behaviors and family empathy, symptoms of depression, feelings of job satisfaction and burnout, and intentions to quit. Of interest were not only the detection of any overall effects of the intervention but also whether the effects of the intervention were stronger for any particular subgroup in the study. For families, we compared family members of residents with and without dementia; for staff, we compared nurses (RNs/LPNs) to CNAs.

The results of the treatment–control comparisons are positive for both staff and family members (Pillemer et al., 2003). The strongest effects were found for both groups' attitudes about the other: Family members on intervention units perceived greater empathy on the part of the staff in both the short and long term following the program, and staff members viewed family behaviors toward them as more positive, particularly in the first 2 months after the workshops. Furthermore, staff members in the treatment group improved in their feelings toward the job, as indicated by a reduction in their predicted likelihood of quitting. Finally, reports of conflict with staff members declined among family members whose relatives had dementia. Nurses and CNAs did not differ in their responses to the program.

Notably, the strongest effects generally were found on the first posttest, with diminishing strength at the 6-month posttest. This suggests that the impact of PIC diminishes over time, perhaps because the skills require additional practice and reinforcement to be maintained. Turnover in residents and staff probably contributes to this pattern as well. This pattern of findings suggests that staff and family members might benefit from the provision of additional "booster sessions" following the initial workshops and at regular intervals thereafter. Because they would occur some weeks after the initial training and could be shorter than the full workshops, the time commitment might not be perceived as burdensome.

These results regarding the outcome measures coincide with overwhelmingly positive subjective evaluations of the PIC intervention by participants. Ninety-eight percent of family members ($n = 323$) and staff members ($n = 256$) reported that they could associate the material covered to their own experiences in the nursing home. Between 82% and 97% of each group reported learning new ways of communicating with each other, increased understanding of the other group's behavior and feelings, and more comfort in voicing concerns. Ninety-two percent of participants rated the program as excellent or good, and 96% reported that they would recommend the program to others in their situations. Such a response is highly encouraging because it suggests that similar interventions are likely to be both welcomed and effective across a range of long-term care settings.

A final contributing indicator of the program's effects takes the form of a qualitative process evaluation that was carried out throughout the project's development. Regular discussions were held with the trainers, and their experiences and suggestions were used to revise the program. In addition, staff and family members were interviewed to learn more about how the program could be improved. Thus, the PIC program is not just the product of a few people but instead has benefited from the insights of trainers, nurses, nursing assistants, family members, and facility administrators.

PARTNERS IN CAREGIVING
IN THE SPECIAL CARE UNIT ENVIRONMENT

The critical next step in developing the PIC program was to broaden its applicability to other long-term care settings. In 2000, Dr. Robison received a grant from the HCR ManorCare Foundation to adapt and pilot-test PIC in SCUs. A multidisciplinary group of dementia care experts collaborated to adapt the PIC training manual for the SCU environment. The basic structure of the program remained similar, but the new version added a module on understanding dementia and related behavioral symptoms and all case studies focused on residents with dementia. Two nursing facilities with SCUs (one for-profit and one not-for-profit) volunteered as pilot sites.

Four months after the PIC-SCU workshops and joint meetings, results demonstrated very positive ratings from staff and families. Participants reported reductions in caregiver burden, in reported hassles with staff, and in reported conflicts with families. Pre- and postworkshop inventories of resident dementia-related behaviors showed improvements in resident behavioral symptoms. Both facilities demonstrated significant changes in facility policies ranging from small (e.g., purchasing special safety name tags for staff and creating "get to know the staff" bulletin boards) to large (hiring new recreational therapy staff and implementing a process for keeping families informed about medical visits and results).

Presently, a controlled-intervention study of the PIC-SCU program is under way in 20 nursing homes with SCUs or dementia programs, funded by a 3-year grant from the Alzheimer's Association to Dr. Robison. This project design parallels that of the evaluation of the original PIC program described previously, with the exception that, because most facilities with dedicated dementia care have only one SCU, there are no control units within intervention facilities. The original PIC evaluation detected no differences between the control units in the intervention facilities and those in the control facilities.

The PIC-SCU intervention includes 20 facilities in three Connecticut counties, randomly selected from all facilities with SCUs. Telephone interviews are conducted with nursing staff and families at the same three time points (baseline and 2 and 6 months later). In addition, facility staff members complete behavioral symptom checklists for all unit residents before and 2 months after the workshops (and at parallel times in the control groups). Finally, qualitative interviews with facility administrators assess their success in meeting the goals established at the joint meeting. Thus, the evaluation goes a few steps beyond the original program's assessment to report effects of the program in both proprietary and not-for-profit facilities and to examine the program's impact on residents and on facility policies and practices. Data collection is still in progress, but program evaluations collected at the close of the workshops indicate high levels of satisfaction, comparable to those reported for the original PIC program. As with the original PIC evaluation, ongoing feedback is solicited from trainers, program participants, and nursing home administrative staff to inform program modifications.

IMPLEMENTING THE
PARTNERS IN CAREGIVING PROGRAMS

The PIC programs seek to improve or prevent strained and conflictual staff–family relationships, which can lead to the alienation of family members and to decreased involvement with their relatives. Specifically, families and the nursing home staff who participate in the program learn how to communicate more effectively with each other, to avoid problems, and to solve problems when they occur. Such improved communication makes it more likely that both parties will work cooperatively to improve the quality of care for residents.

The PIC programs are founded on what has come to be termed an *empowerment* approach. Empowerment programs help people to develop their own skills and work in their own communities. Most relations between families and nursing homes are not based on empowerment; in fact, long-term care arrangements often make both family and staff members feel *powerless* and unable to affect the conditions in which care takes place.

In contrast, an empowerment-oriented program views families and nursing home staff as expert partners. Mutual respect and caring form the basis of this partnership, with families bringing their knowledge of who their relative is, staff members bringing technical expertise in providing quality care, and each caring for the resident with dementia. To this basic partnership, many other valuable insights and skills are added, and a feeling of care between family and staff members develops.

The PIC programs consist of two parallel workshop series: one for family members and one for nursing home staff. The staff workshop is structured as a 5- to 6-hour in-service day. The family program includes one 4- to 5-hour session. This schedule may not be possible for some facilities, and other options are provided. The program ends with a joint session among families, facility staff, and administrators. It is very important that administrators are fully supportive of the project; this final session allows them to become involved and provides them with a unique opportunity to learn how staff and family members perceive the facility.

A PIC team is formed in each facility to plan the implementation of the program in the nursing home. This team usually consists of a combination of the director of social services, a nursing assistant, an involved family member, the director of nursing, a staff development coordinator, and the facility administrator. This group meets to review the basic content of the training and to handle scheduling and logistical issues. By being part of the planning team, administrators show support for the program from the outset.

Three members of this planning team serve as facilitators for the program when it is run in the facility. A common way to run the program utilizes the director of social services, or a designated social worker, as a co-facilitator at both the staff and family workshops. In the staff in-service, a nursing assistant serves as co-facilitator; in the family seminars, a family member of a resident acts as co-facilitator. Staff development personnel also frequently serve as the co-facilitator in both sessions.

Detailed manuals for each PIC program are available for the planning team's and facilitators' use. They are not participant manuals; instead, they provide detailed directions for facilitators who will conduct the training. Ideally, facilitators will attend a "train-the-trainers" session before conducting the program. However, the exercises are described in detail in the manual and provide a good overview of the goals and activities of the project. The original PIC program manual is available for use on non–dementia care units; the PIC-SCU environment manual is available for the dementia care unit setting. Because the contents of the two versions of the program are very similar, program details contained in this chapter apply to both versions, unless otherwise specified.

The contents of the staff and family sessions are nearly identical. The major difference is in the specific case studies used for discussion. However, the basic communication skills learned are the same. Before running the workshops, a facilitator needs to carefully review both the staff and family versions of the exercises to note some important differences in wording.

Program Components

The components of the PIC program are arranged in an order that allows later units to build on earlier ones (Table 9.1). Thus, the program begins with an introduction to PIC and a chance for the participants to introduce themselves. In the PIC-SCU version, a group discussion of dementia and related behavioral symptoms follows. The next unit ("Sharing Successful Family–Staff Communication") lets the group members get some of their concerns out in the open but also focuses on positive aspects of the facility. The next two sections ("Advanced Listening Skills" and "Saying What You Mean Clearly and Respectfully") cover communication and active listening techniques.

The following three units deal with situations in which cooperative communication is particularly difficult in the nursing home: when there are cultural and ethnic barriers to communication; when values among different groups in the facility affect communication; and when a person must deal with blame, criticism, and conflict. (The final component of the program, a joint session with administrators, is discussed later.)

The manual contains a number of exercises and techniques to involve participants in learning new skills. PIC is not a didactic program,

Table 9.1. Components of the Partners in Caregiving workshop

Introduction to Partners in Caregiving: The theoretical background and goals of the program are introduced, with a brief warm-up introduction exercise for participants.

Sharing successful family-staff communication: The group participates in a brainstorming exercise in which they share concerns about communicating with the other group. A list of positive aspects of communication within the facility is also generated.

Advanced listening skills: In this interactive skill-building session, participants learn active listening skills, feedback techniques, and how to avoid "communication blockers."

Saying what you mean clearly and respectfully: The concept of "I-messages" is explored, using role-playing exercises to learn how to put them into practice.

Cultural and ethnic differences: The concepts of cultural and ethnic diversity in the facility are introduced, with discussion of how these concepts can affect good communication.

Handling blame, criticism, and conflict: A seven-step process for preventing and dealing with conflict with the other group is discussed. Techniques are practiced using role play and case study approaches.

Understanding differences in values: Participants explore differences in values of various groups in the nursing home (family, staff, administration, residents). Differences in values and their impact are discussed.

Planning a joint session for families, staff, and administrators: Group members plan, organize, and develop an agenda for a joint meeting.

Joint session (2 hours): Both groups meet to share what they have learned and discuss their concerns with the administrator. A plan is developed to identify policy and procedural changes and address them as a team

although information is sometimes given to participants in lecture form. Instead, the program is one in which participants learn and practice new skills. The program will be successful to the extent that the facilitators can get the group actively involved in the learning process. Because this is not always an easy task, PIC contains a number of structured exercises and role plays in which group members actually use what they have learned.

A number of case studies are presented in the manual (sometimes in the context of role plays). An example is the discussion of the "conflict resolution script" in the section titled "Handling Blame, Criticism, and Conflict." Case discussions take abstract concepts and make them concrete. A major goal is to identify how the communication techniques learned in PIC could have a positive effect on the case. The facilitators' role in case discussions is to encourage participants to react and to keep the discussion open and nonjudgmental.

The manual provides a number of pages that can be duplicated as handouts and made into overhead transparencies (these appear at the end of the manual). Showing an overhead helps focus the group's attention on what is being discussed, and individuals with vision problems or reading difficulties will appreciate having a copy as well. The handouts also serve as reference materials that can be reviewed at home. Therefore, each participant receives a complete set of the handouts.

Because no two facilities are exactly alike, PIC stresses flexibility. For example, in the nursing homes in which PIC was evaluated, it was clear that some exercises worked better than others in various facilities and that some training schedules were more appropriate than others. Therefore, as a training team becomes more familiar with PIC, they not only can but also *should* adapt and individualize the program to meet the needs and challenges within their given settings.

Training Components

Four basic types of training components are used in the PIC programs: minilectures, brainstorming, small-group discussions, and role plays.

Minilectures

At various points in the manual, the trainer is directed to give a short talk about a topic. An example is the "Introduction to Partners in Caregiving" unit that appears at the beginning of both the family and staff trainings. These "minilectures" are printed in bold type in the manual, and they are intended to convey basic knowledge and information to the participants. However, these minilectures are not designed to be read word-for-word out of the manual. Trainers should familiarize themselves with the content of each minilecture and make it their own. A good idea is to personalize the minilectures by adding examples from one's own facility.

Brainstorming

In these exercises, participants generate ideas about a topic in a free, open discussion. An example is the "Sharing Successful Family–Staff Communication" unit in which participants note factors that both encourage and discourage communication. The goal of a brainstorming exercise is to collect ideas from as many group members as possible. These ideas are not immediately judged or evaluated as good or bad; they are listed on newsprint or a blackboard for later group discussion. The trainer's role is to be encouraging and positive, to assure the group that there are no "right" answers, and to summarize and draw connections among the various comments.

Small-Group Discussions

At some points in the program, the larger group is divided into several smaller ones. An example is in the unit on "Cultural and Ethnic Differences," in which small groups discuss questions about this topic. A major function of the small groups is to allow and encourage reticent members of the group to express their ideas. Some people may be uncomfortable sharing their ideas in a group of 12 but find it easy to do so in a group of 3 or 4. This is especially true when sensitive topics are discussed. At the end of a small-group exercise, each group reports on the main points raised in its discussion.

Role Plays

Although some people are resistant to role playing, in PIC it was found that there is simply no better alternative for learning and practicing the skills highlighted in the program. Participants in role plays have the opportunity to try out a new technique in a structured, "safe" setting. Even if a group member is not one of the role players, he or she benefits by seeing the technique "in action." Suggestions for how to facilitate role plays are provided in the manuals' appendices.

GUIDELINES FOR PLANNING AND CONDUCTING PARTNERS IN CAREGIVING

Based on evaluations of PIC, the authors of this chapter have learned a considerable amount about what works and what does not when implementing the program. Accordingly, the authors have developed general guidelines on how to plan for and conduct PIC.

Step 1: Create a Partners in Caregiving Planning Group

The most important step is to organize a planning group in each facility that will guide PIC through its development and implementation. This group should include, at a minimum, the facility administrator, the director of social services, the director of nursing, a nursing assistant, and a family member. Getting a group such as this together may be difficult, but it is one of the most important parts of PIC, for two reasons. First, the planning group represents the initial step in improving family–staff relations. By discussing the training issues and planning the program, administrators, staff, and family members begin the process of learning to work together in new ways. Second, support from the facility administration is key to the success of the program; in our evaluation, those facilities that had supportive, involved administrators had a more successful experience, especially in the joint meeting at the end of the program.

It may not be possible for the entire planning group to meet as a whole throughout the course of the project. At a bare minimum, it is critical that at least one meeting be held with the administrator during the planning stages and that he or she receive regular updates throughout the project. Because one possible outcome of the program is change in administrative policies, the need for administrator involvement is obvious.

The planning group's first task is to familiarize itself with the PIC programs. Members should read the manuals, and one or more members should attend a train-the-trainers program if available. These programs are periodically sponsored by Cornell University and can be arranged upon request by a group of nursing homes. (For more information, please see the Resources section at the end of the chapter.)

Second, the planning group will need to make a series of decisions throughout the planning process. These decisions include 1) creating a training team; 2) deciding on who should be invited to participate in the program; 3) figuring out logistics, such as location and time of the training; and 4) selecting the person responsible for arrangements.

Step 2: Create a Training Team

The first major decision of the planning group will be deciding who will conduct the training. The selection of facilitators is very important. Indeed, the authors of this chapter learned in their evaluation that the facilitator's approach and comfort level had a major impact on the success of the program. The members of the training team should also become members of the planning group and meet with it regularly.

In establishing the training team, an important decision is whether to use an internal or external facilitator. In the authors' projects, facilitators have included social workers employed by the nursing home (in the smaller facilities, this was the director of social services; in larger facilities, a member of the social work staff) and trainers hired by the researchers, all of whom had extensive group leadership experience.

There are several advantages to using an internal facilitator. First, he or she has an intimate knowledge of the nursing home, its residents, and its policies. Second, he or she can provide continuity after the training and can help to implement changes identified by families and staff. Third, because it may otherwise be necessary to hire an outside facilitator, using a current staff member can provide savings to the facility.

In contrast, a major advantage to using an outside facilitator is that both staff and family members may be more open with an "outsider." Staff members may fear that problems they raise will somehow "get back" to the administration and cause them (the staff) to be negatively evaluated. Family members may be afraid of seeming to be "complainers." Also, in a few cases, facilitators from within the nursing home became uncomfortable conducting role plays and other exercises with their co-workers. Sometimes, an outsider is able to take more risks and persuade participants—in a way that a staff member cannot—to try something new.

Who are potential outside facilitators? Local social workers or psychologists are certainly possibilities. A particularly good option may be a former employee of the nursing home (e.g., a social worker) who has left for reasons such as retirement or the birth of a child, but who would be interested in serving as a trainer on a part-time basis. Such a person combines knowledge of the facility with an "outsider" status. Another possibility in some states is Cooperative Extension agents, an increasing number of whom are becoming knowledgeable in issues of aging. A third option is to work in partnership with a neighboring nursing home and switch social work staff for training. This option offers a no-cost "outside consultant."

Based on experience, the authors of this chapter anticipate that most facilities will use a member of their social work staff or staff development personnel to conduct the training. The authors' evaluation shows that this is usually very successful and that the trainers become even better at conducting the workshops as they become more experienced at it. However, as the authors have stated previously, the key is flexibility—for example, trying the program first with the facility social worker as the trainer and then with an outside trainer the second time.

In addition to the facilitator, the training team for PIC includes two co-facilitators: ideally, a nursing assistant and a family member. The facilitator conducts the staff training with the nursing assistant as the co-facilitator and the family training with the family member as co-facilitator. The co-facilitators are very important to the success of the training. The first reason relates to the empowerment model. It is extremely empowering for group members when "one of their own," so to speak, acts as a trainer. The training then takes place on a more equal level and makes it clear that the knowledge of the participants is what the training is all about. Second, on a more practical level, conducting PIC, although rewarding, can also at times be somewhat stressful; it is much better to share the responsibility with someone else. Third, serving as a co-facilitator can improve the self-esteem and empowerment of the nursing assistants and family members themselves.

Step 3: Select a Unit for the Training

Although this may differ from facility to facility, the authors of this chapter strongly recommend that PIC be conducted on a unit-by-unit basis. That is, rather than selecting families and staff from the entire facility, it may be more effective to concentrate on training the staff and families on one unit at one time. This way, families and staff members have a common frame of reference and learn the same skills. It is also often easier to try out changes in policies on a single unit. If a dementia SCU is selected, facilitators should utilize the PIC-SCU version of the manual for the training.

Step 4: Select and Recruit Participants

If possible, it is best that the training be made available to all interested staff and family members on a unit. Because the optimal size for a training group is between 8 and 12 participants, to maintain adequate staffing on the unit during the staff workshop time it may be necessary to conduct more than one training. Of course, it is unlikely that all members of either group will be able to take part, but it has been the chapter authors' experience in PIC that, when even a few family and staff members on a unit go through the program, there is a "ripple effect" as the participants share the skills they have learned with others.

Initial recruitment for PIC is not likely to be a major problem. In the authors' experience, both staff and family members are very interested and eager to take part in programs such as this. Promotional letters that the chapter authors developed for the project appear in the manuals' appendices.

Two special recruitment decisions must be made in terms of the staff. First, the question arises: Who should be trained? In the authors' sites, both nurses and nursing assistants were trained together in a single group. The authors made this decision because they felt that the program would also help improve nurse–nursing assistant communication and solidarity. In general, this worked very well, and very few negative comments were received in the evaluation. A facility may wish to include other staff members who have frequent contact with families as well.

The second decision relates to payment of staff for the time spent in the training. Although some staff members may consent to take part in the training on their own time, we strongly suggest that staff members receive their regular wage during the training. Obviously, for some staff members this may be the only way they can participate, but for all staff, receiving payment for the training demonstrates the administration's commitment to improving communication in the facility. Some facilities may choose to use PIC as part of their regular in-service education for staff. This approach would integrate the program into the nursing home philosophy.

Step 5: Prepare Training

The first time a new training program is started, it is always a challenge. The key to success with PIC is preparation and rehearsal. The more familiar that trainers become with the materials, the better the trainers' and participants' experiences will be.

The co-facilitators should carefully read the materials in the manual. A decision must then be made about the roles each co-facilitator will play. They should decide among themselves who will lead each exercise, who will keep an eye on the time, who will handle the overhead transparencies or slides, and so forth.

A key point to remember is this: Different people have differing levels of comfort leading trainings. Co-facilitators may decide, for example, that one person will do most of the talking to the entire group and the other will lead some of the exercises. Another facilitator may not feel comfortable leading role plays but may be happy to do the minilectures. There is no right and wrong here; the goal is both to demonstrate how people can work well together and to relieve the pressure on a single facilitator.

A clear key to success is to rehearse all training components. A good idea is to ask members of the planning group to take part in a "dry run" of the exercises. This allows the facilitators to practice and also helps the planning team learn what PIC is all about. It is important that the facilitators not go into the training "cold." The better they know the materials and the more practice they have had with them, the more successful the training will be.

Step 6: Time, Location, and Arrangements

Based on the evaluation, the authors of this chapter believe that the most effective schedule for PIC is a 5- to 6-hour in-service for staff members and one 4- to 5-hour workshop for family members. (The 2-hour joint session for staff, family, and administrators takes place after both groups are finished). However, some sites had two or three sessions for the staff and found that this also worked well. It is not recommended, however, that the training be provided in four or more sessions over a month or more. Because each section builds on the previous one, if the gap between the first and last session is too long, knowledge will be lost. The chance that participants will drop out also increases as more sessions are added.

For reasons of convenience and cost, many facilities will choose to conduct PIC on site. This has the advantage that participants will not have difficulty finding the training location. However, a different site gets people out of the nursing home setting, where they may feel more open to new ideas and have a greater sense of confidentiality. Facilities may wish to experiment with the location.

One consideration that relates to both time and location is the reluctance of some family elders to travel at night. However, holding the training during the day excludes working family members. If sessions are to be held in the evening, they should be held as early as possible. For example, a family member training session could take place at 5:30 P.M., with a break for a simple dinner. Another option is to have two family training groups, one during the day and one in the evening; this allows a maximum number of family members to participate. Regardless of when the training is held, serving light refreshments (or lunch or dinner, depending on the timing of the training) is strongly suggested. Sharing food often makes a group more cohesive and provides the opportunity for informal communication during a break in the training.

Step 7: The Joint Session

After both staff and family members have completed the training, a joint session is held with all of the training participants and the administrator. The joint session is the culmination of the PIC program. It can be an extremely empowering experience for family and staff members, one that greatly increases their understanding for one another. As noted earlier, the session can also result in concrete changes in facility practice or policy that make both staff and family members happier. However, trainers may have concerns that this session may become overly confrontational or that it will turn into a "gripe session."

There are several keys to the success of the joint session. One is anticipating in advance the problematic topics that may arise and meeting with the administrator to prepare him or her for the session. The role of the administrator is to listen to the staff and family members and to brainstorm solutions with them. He or she must be open to the participants' suggestions and must try not to react defensively. Another key is for the facilities to remind participants to use some of the communication skills they learned in the training session. The co-trainers must play an active role in keeping the discussion on a productive and nonconfrontational level.

Facilities may want to experiment with the joint session and develop a format that works best for them. One suggestion that arose from an evaluation was to hold two joint sessions. The first would involve just the family and staff training participants, to let them get to know one another and to plan the meeting with the administrator together. The administrator would then be invited to the second session.

The joint session closes with informal discussion among the participants over refreshments. It presents a rare opportunity for family members, staff members, and administrators to step back from the daily ongoing stress of the unit and discuss ways to improve resident care and encourage family involvement. In many cases, it becomes clear that problem issues for families result from *lack of knowledge* about institutional policies rather than problems with the policies themselves. In these situations, it is relatively easy for administrative staff, with input from other staff and family members themselves, to set goals to remedy the difficulties discussed during the joint meeting.

Within a few days after the joint meeting, PIC facilitators organize the notes from the meeting into issues raised and goals set and distribute the document to all unit staff members, all family members (including those who did not participate in the trainings), and residents where appropriate. When the time period to accomplish the stated goals expires, the facilitators complete their final task of assessing which goals have been met and describing ongoing plans related to issues discussed at the joint meeting.

CONCLUSION

The Partners in Caregiving and Partners in Caregiving in a Special Care Unit environment programs represent the culmination of many years of development and evaluation. Extension of the PIC program continues with the ongoing evaluation of the PIC-SCU program, the development of Caring Communication (a program for staff and families focused on end-of-life issues), and planned adaptations for assisted living, home care, and other long-term care settings. The Caring Communication program emphasizes communication processes aimed at improving end-of-life care by facilitating more positive relations between family and staff members. The program consists of two parallel workshop series: one for family members and one for nursing home staff. The staff workshop is structured as two 2-hour segments. The family program consists of a 1-hour workshop that can be worked into a family council meeting. The program also includes a booster session, designed to occur a month or more after the initial in-service training. Evaluation results of each PIC program show high participant satisfaction, lasting change in staff and family attitudes and behaviors, and an impact on policies and practices in nursing homes that affect family involvement.

REFERENCES

Bauer, M., & Nay, R. (2003). Family and staff partnerships in long-term care: A review of the literature. *Journal of Gerontological Nursing, 29*(10), 46–53.

Caris-Vehallen, W., Kerkstra, A., & Bensing, J.M. (1997). The role of communication in nursing care for elderly people: A review of the literature. *Journal of Advanced Nursing, 27,* 915–933.

Cochran, M., & Dean, C. (1991). Home–school relations and the empowerment process. *The Elementary School Journal, 91,* 261–269.

Cohen-Mansfield, J. (1995). Stress in nursing home staff: A review and a theoretical model. *Journal of Applied Gerontology, 14,* 444–466.

Davis, L.L., & Buckwalter, K. (2001). Family caregiving after nursing home admission. *Journal of Mental Health & Aging, 7,* 361–369.

Duncan, M.T., & Morgan, D.L. (1994). Sharing the caring: Family caregivers' views of their relationships with nursing home staff. *The Gerontologist, 34,* 235–244.

Ekman, S.L., & Norberg, A. (1988). The autonomy of demented patients: Interviews with caregivers. *Journal of Medical Ethics, 14,* 184–187.

Gaugler, J.E., Andersen, K.A., Zarit, S.H., & Pearlin, L.I. (2004). Family involvement in nursing homes: Effects on stress and well-being. *Aging & Mental Health, 8,* 65–75.

George, L.K., & Maddox, G.L. (1989). Social behavior aspects of institutional care. In M.G. Ory & K. Bond (Eds.), *Aging and health care: Social science and policy perspectives* (pp. 116–141). New York: Routledge.

Greenberg, J.M., Doblin, B.H., Shapiro, D.W., Linn, L.S., & Wenger, N.S. (1993). Effect of an educational program on medical students' conversations with patients about advance directives: A randomized trial. *Journal of General Internal Medicine, 8,* 683–685.

Greene, V., & Monahan, D. (1982). The impact of visitation on patient well-being in nursing homes. *The Gerontologist, 22,* 418–423.

Heiselman, T., & Noelker, L.S. (1991). Enhancing mutual respect among nursing assistants, residents, and residents' families. *The Gerontologist, 31,* 552–555.

Henderson, A.T., & Berla, N. (Eds.). (1994). *A new generation of evidence: The family is critical to student achievement.* Washington, DC: National Committee for Citizens in Education.

Hertzberg, A., & Ekman, S.L. (1996). How the relatives of elderly patients in institutional care perceive the staff. *Scandinavian Journal of Caring Sciences, 10,* 205–211.

Krause, A.M., Grant, L.D., & Long, B.C. (1999). Sources of stress reported by daughters of nursing home residents. *Journal of Aging Studies, 13,* 349–364.

Levinson, W., & Roter, D. (1993). The effects of two continuing medical education programs on communication skills of practicing primary care physicians. *Journal of General Internal Medicine, 8,* 318–324.

Litwak, E. (1985). *Helping the elderly: The complimentary roles of informal networks and informal systems.* New York: Guilford.

Litwak, E., Jessop, D.J., & Moulton, H.J. (1994). Optimal use of formal and informal systems over the life course. In E. Kahana, D.E. Biegel, & M.L. Wykle (Eds.), *Family caregiver application series: Vol. 1. Family caregiving across the lifespan* (pp. 96–130). Thousand Oaks, CA: Sage.

Logue, R.M. (2003). Maintaining family connectedness in long-term care: An advanced practice approach to family-centered nursing homes. *Journal of Gerontological Nursing, 29*(6), 24–31.

McCormick, W.C., Inui, T.S., & Roter, D.L. (1996). Interventions in physician–elderly patient interactions. *Research on Aging, 18,* 103–136.

Noelker, L., & Harel, Z. (1978). Predictors of well-being and survival among institutionalized aged. *The Gerontologist, 18,* 562–567.

Nolan, M., & Dellasega, C. (1999). It's not the same as him being home: Creating caring partnerships following nursing home placement. *Journal of Clinical Nursing, 8,* 723–730.

Peak, T. (2000). Families and the nursing home environment: Adaptation in a group context. *Journal of Gerontological Social Work, 33,* 51–66.

Penrod, J.D., Kane, R.A., & Kane, R.L. (2000). Effects of post-hospital informal care on nursing home discharge. *Research on Aging, 22,* 66–82.

Pillemer, K. (1996). *Solving the frontline crisis in long-term care.* Cambridge, MA: Frontline Publishing.

Pillemer, K., Hegeman, C.R., Albright, B., & Henderson, C. (1998). Building bridges between families and nursing home staff: The Partners in Caregiving program. *The Gerontologist, 38,* 499–503.

Pillemer, K., Suitor, J.J., Henderson, C.R., Meador, R., Schultz, L., Robison, J., et al. (2003). A cooperative communication intervention for nursing home staff and family members of residents. *The Gerontologist, 43*(Special issue 2), 96–106.

Safford, F. (1989). If you don't like the care, why don't you take your mother home? Obstacles to family/staff partnerships in the institutional care of the aged. *Journal of Gerontological Social Work, 13,* 1–7.

Specht, J.P., Kelley, L.S., Manion, P., Maas, M.L., Reed, D., & Rantz, M.J. (2000). Who's the boss? Family/staff partnership in care of persons with dementia. *Nursing Administration Quarterly, 24,* 64–77.

Stephens, M.A.P., Ogrocki, P.K., & Kinney, J.K. (1991). Sources of stress for family caregivers of institutionalized dementia patients. *Journal of Applied Gerontology, 10,* 328–342.

Stull, D.E., Cosbey, J., Bowman, K., & McNutt, W. (1997). Institutionalization: A continuation of family care. *Journal of Applied Gerontology, 16,* 379–402.

Tobin, S. (1995). Fostering family involvement in institutional care. In G.C. Smith, S.S. Tobin, E.A. Robertson-Tchabo, & P.W. Power (Eds.), *Strengthening aging families: Diversity in practice and policy* (pp. 25–44). Thousand Oaks, CA: Sage.

Tornatore, J.B., & Grant, L.A. (2004). Family caregiver satisfaction with the nursing home after placement of a relative with dementia. *Journals of Gerontology. Series B, Psychological Sciences and Social Sciences, 59,* S80–S88.

RESOURCES

The program manuals developed for PIC facilitators provide detailed instructions and necessary materials for implementing the programs. The chapter authors strongly recommend implementing the program on a regular basis either in full or with shorter booster sessions highlighting different sections of the workshop. By design, family turnover regularly occurs in nursing homes, as residents move in and out. In addition, high staff turnover rates in nursing homes require continuing opportunities for training on how to communicate effectively with family members to engage them as full partners in the care of their relatives.

The Cornell Institute for Translational Research on Aging or the Center on Aging at the University of Connecticut Health Center can provide technical assistance and trainers for implementing the PIC project. Options include customized training for single facilities and train-the-trainer sessions for small teams and large groups. A manual can also be purchased. For information on the training or to order a manual, please contact

Rhoda Meador
Cornell Institute for Translational Research on Aging
Beebe Hall
Cornell University
Ithaca, NY 14853
E mail: rhm2@cornell.edu
Telephone: 607-254-5360
Fax: 607-254-2903

For information on the PIC-SCU program or to order a manual, please contact

Julie Robison, Ph.D.
University of Connecticut Health Center
Center on Aging
263 Farmington Avenue
Farmington, CT 06030-6147
E-mail: jrobison@uchc.edu
Telephone: 860-679-4278
Fax: 860-679-8023

For information on the Caring Communication program or to order a manual, please contact

Carol Hegeman
Director of Research
Foundation for Long Term Care
150 State Street
Albany, NY 12207
E-mail: chegeman@nyahsa.org
Telephone: 518-449-7873, ext. 125
Fax: 518-434-4385

For information about the topics covered in this chapter, please contact

Karl A. Pillemer, Ph.D.
Professor, Human Development

Cornell University
G44 Martha Van Rensselaer Hall
Ithaca, NY 14853
E-mail: kap6@cornell.edu
Telephone: 607-255-8086
Fax: 607-255-8767

IV

The Future of Family Involvement Interventions

10

Educating Families and Improving Communication

A Web-Based Intervention Program for Families of Nursing Home Residents with Dementia

VALERIE E. TOLBERT AND JENNIFER G. BASHAM

In 2000, an estimated 4.5 million Americans were living with Alzheimer's disease (Herbert, Scherr, Bienias, Bennett, & Evans, 2003). Because of the aging of the population, the number of Americans with this and other dementias is expected to increase in the coming years. Most family members are able to care for their relatives at home initially, but, as symptoms worsen, many must admit their relatives to nursing homes. After admitting a relative to a nursing home, most families continue their commitment to the caregiver role (Duncan & Morgan, 1994; Keefe & Fancey, 2000; Murphy et al., 2000). Many family members report feeling relieved that the burden of daily care has been lifted but also report an increased emotional burden of guilt (Ryan & Scullion, 2000). Families often report that it is difficult for them to stay involved and to continue to provide support. Some of these difficulties are due to restricted opportunities to visit because family members may live far away or may have limited time. Other family members report that it is challenging to plan visits around the daily routines conducted in nursing homes. Previous research has shown that family members often have unrealistic expectations of the care and services that can be provided in a nursing home (McAfee, 1999). Families want quality care and quality environments for their relatives but have a hard time accepting that *any* nursing home can provide what they want (Grau, Teresi, Burton, & Chandler, 1995; McAfee, 1999). As a result, some family members criticize the care their relatives are receiving and find the perceived inflexibility of staff and daily routines irritating. Family members' dissatisfaction can disrupt a resident's adjustment to life in a nursing home, so improving family members' satisfaction with nursing home care can be an important area for intervention.

Because of families' unrealistic expectations and the very different roles they play in providing care, family members and the administration and staff of nursing homes sometimes develop adversarial relationships. The development of adversarial exchange can be predicted by a theoretical framework that has been applied to various social relationships—for example, conflicts that arise in informal networks embedded within more formal organizations. In this particular instance, the formal organization is the nursing home and the informal embedded network is the family (Rosen et al., 2003). Both the nursing home and the family share the responsibility of optimizing resident comfort, care, and safety.

The philosophy and techniques of formal and informal networks differ greatly. For example, the administration and the staff use established policies and procedures. Decisions are made using medical science or possibly based on financial concern. Residents are constantly monitored, and their physical and mental health is always being assessed. Nursing home staff members are legally required to provide a safe and therapeutic environment and must meet state and federal standards for safety. Nursing homes are regularly inspected and monitored by state departments of health and other regulatory agencies to ensure that they are in compliance with these standards (Stevenson et al., 2000). The bureaucracy required in the long-term care system means that subjectivity is reduced and standardization of care becomes common.

In contrast, family members interact with residents in very different ways. Family members typically are not present most of the time and typically are not trained to monitor their relatives in a professional way. They may provide some hands-on care, but many of their interactions are social in nature. Families have a prior knowledge of residents that is typically unavailable to the nursing home staff. They may perceive the resident as deteriorating more quickly than do staff members, who may have a different baseline expectation of the resident's behavior and health. Families tend to want personalized, individualized treatment for their relatives. Family opinions and attitude are important to the resident's quality of life because families often influence or actually make decisions for the resident (Binstock & Spector, 1997). Families need adequate knowledge about dementia and the routines of the nursing home to make such decisions.

The potential for conflict between the formal organization (the nursing home) and the informal network (the family) is high (Weber, 1947). Families tend to view nursing home staff caregivers and their routines as mechanistic and insensitive. The staff, in turn, may undervalue the importance of family input, observation, and opinion. If conflict between the formal and informal network is not addressed, less-than-optimal care for the resident may be the result.

Some researchers have suggested that a model of "shared functions" could bring formal and informal networks together and provide better care for residents (Litwak & Figuiera, 1970; Sussman, 1977). This model suggests multiple components to resident care. Some aspects of care are best handled by the nursing home staff, whereas others are best handled by the family. In order for this model to work, families must be familiar with what the staff members do and can do for their residents. Unfortunately, current research suggests that families lack some basic knowledge about the routines and procedures conducted by nursing home staff. They also lack knowledge about ways they can be involved to improve the care of their relatives.

INTERVENTIONS TO IMPROVE
FAMILY–STAFF INTERACTIONS

Several researchers have noted the need to bring staff and family members together, and several interventions have been designed to improve family–staff communications (Boise & White, 2004; Hertzberg & Ekman, 2000; Hertzberg, Ekman, & Axelsson, 2003; Logue, 2003; Marquis, Freegard, & Hoogland, 2004). Some have been shown to be beneficial in specific ways. For example, the Family Involvement in Care intervention improves family emotional reaction to the caregiving role, family perceptions of relationships with staff members, family perception of care for relatives, and the staff's perception of the family caregiving role (Maas et al., 2004; see Chapter 8). Partners in Caregiving (Pillemer, Hegeman, Albright, & Henderson, 1998; Pillemer et al., 2003; see Chapter 9) improved staff and family attitudes toward each other, reduced family–staff conflict, and reduced likelihood of staff turnover. It must be emphasized that simply increasing family–staff interaction and communication with residents can have profound effects on the residents' quality of life. Person-centered communication and feelings of interpersonal closeness have been shown to sometimes increase lucidity, even in people with severe dementia (Normann, Asplund, & Norberg, 1998). Nursing home residents' quality of life can be similarly improved by increasing positive, caring interactions.

Web-based interventions, or telemedicine, may be particularly useful for improving family–staff interactions. *Telemedicine* is defined as a process that uses technology (e.g., telephones, the Internet, multimedia) to support medical and psychosocial care (Ferguson, Doarn, & Scott, 1995). Currently, web-based health education sites and web-based psychosocial interventions exist for many disorders. More than 100,000 health information web sites have been developed that deliver basic information on a variety of health-related problems (Kolata, 2000; Ritterband et al., 2003). Numerous web-based interventions have been developed, including those dealing with issues such as diabetes management (McKay, Glascow, Feil, Boles, & Barrera, 2002), posttraumatic stress disorder and pathological grief (Lange, van de Ven, Schrieken, & Emmelkamp, 2001), weight loss (Tate, Wing, & Winett, 2001; Winett et al., 1999), and panic disorder (Klein & Richards, 2001). Web-based interventions and telehealth interventions appear to offer significant benefits to both users and providers. Some of these benefits include increased access to health services, cost-effectiveness, enhanced educational opportunities, improved health outcomes, better quality of care, better quality of life, and enhanced social support (Jennett, Yeo, Pauls, & Graham, 2003).

ISSUES IN IMPLEMENTING WEB-BASED INTERVENTIONS

Some characteristics make web-based interventions particularly attractive for family members of nursing home residents. The Internet combines attributes of mass communication with attributes of interpersonal communication. General information that is applicable to a majority of people can be provided, as well as specific information or suggestions for individual users. Use of the Internet is convenient and flexible. Family members can participate from wherever they have Internet access (often their homes or offices), eliminating the need for a physical meeting place and the need for participants to travel to that site (Finn, 1995; Weinberg, Uken, Schmale, & Adamek, 1995; Winzelberg, 1997). This can be especially useful for rural patients and their families (Buckwalter, Davis, Wakefield, Kienzle, & Murray, 2002) because opportunities for face-to-face visits may be rare.

The relative anonymity of Internet interactions also can be a positive characteristic. Some evidence suggests that people find it easier to discuss some problems on-line, rather than face-to-face (Kummervold, Gammon, Bergvik, Johnsen, Hasvold, & Rosenvingen, 2002). Finally, family members can participate whenever they have time, usually 24 hours a day, 7 days a week (Liss, Glueckauf, & Ecklund-Johnson, 2002).

Developing Internet interventions is not an easy task. It is time consuming and requires a multidisciplinary team of clinicians and computer experts (e.g., web designers, web graphic artists, computer hardware and software technicians, web programmers). Legal and ethical issues must be considered, including privacy and confidentiality, data validity, and disparities in access to the Internet (Jerome et al., 2000; Koocher & Morray, 2000; Sampson, Kolodinsky, & Greeno, 1997; Winker et al., 2000). A good resource for exploring these issues is the American Medical Association's guidelines for medical and health information sites on the web (Winker et al., 2000; see also Resources section at the end of this chapter). Some factors to consider before deciding to develop a web-based intervention are briefly outlined in the following sections.

Internal Considerations

Extensive planning must occur before the intervention is implemented (Guilfoyle et al., 2002; Hailey & Crowe, 2003). A needs assessment and analysis should be conducted to determine what services are needed (Jennett et al., 2003). A business plan needs to be developed. Management and staff must agree on the need for a telehealth intervention and may require education about the intervention. For telehealth interventions to work effectively, a certain level of stability in management and staff is needed to at least maintain the Internet-based program, which may be difficult in many facilities where staff turnover is extensive.

Liability Issues

Nursing homes and individual providers should consult with a professional liability insurance carrier to ascertain which of the planned services will be covered. Ideally, a written confirmation from the carrier should be obtained (Koocher & Morray, 2000). Users should give informed consent before gaining access to the system, and they must also be adequately trained in the use of the technology to avoid further liability (Britton, 2003; Hogue, 2003).

Confidentiality and Privacy

Internet users rank personal privacy as their most important concern (Winker et al., 2003). The first step in protecting privacy is using the best technology currently available (e.g., firewalls) to prevent unintended access to private information. The American Medical Association requires that personal privacy and confidentiality be respected for both formal (e.g., web pages providing health-related information) and informal (e.g., chat rooms, e-mail, bulletin boards) communications. A careful statement of the limits of confidentiality must be made (Koocher & Morray, 2000). The statement should inform users of the standard limitations to confidentiality (e.g., abuse reporting mandates) and to any existing state-specific limitations. Users must understand that information they provide in informal contexts, such as in chat rooms, may be linked with an identifier, such as a screen name. Users should also be cautioned about privacy problems with broadcast conversations.

Choice of Web Developer

Deciding which web developer to use, if any, is very important. In part, the choice of web developer will determine the services provided and the cost of the intervention. Furthermore, the skill and responsiveness of a web developer can have a serious impact on the success or failure of the intervention. For example, researchers have found that, if the technology did not work the first time a user logged on, acceptance of the technology by users was low (Kobb, Hilsen, & Ryan, 2003). This effect can be mitigated somewhat by educating users about potential problems and troubleshooting strategies. Users should be prepared in advance for technological difficulties and be reassured that any technology-related problems will be promptly resolved. It is important to be aware that agencies and the vendors they use are accountable for correcting technological problems quickly; otherwise, they are potentially liable for breach of care (Hogue, 2003; McCrossin, 2003). Reliability of the technology and the vendor are important factors in the success or failure of web-based interventions (Hailey & Crowe, 2003).

Cost-Effectiveness

Cost-effectiveness must be considered carefully. Most of the cost of the intervention will be related to site development, but there are some ongoing costs for providing access to a web page. The technology and the equipment that make telehealth interventions possible are not inexpensive. The number and type of services offered may depend on the number of likely users. In general, cost is reduced as users are added.

Unfortunately, the assessment of cost-effectiveness is complex and some benefits are likely to remain relatively intangible, such as improved satisfaction with care. Cost-effectiveness must also be considered from multiple perspectives, including those of the resident, the family, the staff, the administration, and payers/insurers (Hailey & Jennett, 2004). Several methods of estimating cost-effectiveness have been proposed, including social audit analysis (Crowe, Hailey, & Carter, 1992) and a cost–consequences matrix (McIntosh & Cairns, 1997). Informal measures can also be developed and used.

Limited Computer Experience of Potential Users

Many older adults have limited experience with computers and may exhibit resistance and suspicion (Trentin, 2004). Research from several studies on Internet interventions suggests that even individuals who are unfamiliar with technology are able to use it with minimal training and have been shown to benefit from the intervention (e.g., McKay et al., 2002). Some specific strategies for teaching older adults about computers and the Internet have been identified (e.g., Hendrix & Sakauye, 2001). Older adults who have learned to use the Internet are successfully finding health-related information, communicating with family members, and expanding their social networks by participating in chat rooms, forums, and bulletin boards (Adams, Oye, & Parker, 2003; Scanlon, 2001).

The complexity of web-based services relies, in part, on the computer literacy of the users. Some older people are avid users of the Internet. Research shows that Internet use (Morrell, 2002a) and computer sales are growing most quickly for adults older than 60 years (Conover, 1997). Other older adults have limited experience with computers or no experience at all. Some opportunities for computer training should be available for unskilled users. For many nonusers, simply learning about how to use a computer can be empowering. Developing skills in computer literacy provides an opportunity for personal growth for older people but also offers the possibility of providing them with a range of network-based systems outside of a computer-based family intervention itself (Irizarry & Downing, 1997; Trentin, 2004). Information can be provided about health and aging, and interactive services can offer an opportunity to consult experts or peers about life choices.

Physical and Cognitive Limitations of Potential Users

Empirical studies have shown some very important differences between people with functional impairments, such as older adults with disabilities, and functionally independent people when they interact with computers (Keats, Langdon, Clarkson, & Robinson, 2002). Currently, most health-related web sites are not accessible by people with disabilities (Davis, 2002). Some limitations commonly experienced by older adults are physical (e.g., difficulty seeing the cursor on the screen, difficulty manipulating the mouse because of arthritis or other conditions). Other limitations are due to cognitive challenges (e.g., difficulty remembering passwords, problems mastering new and unfamiliar vocabulary). Fortunately, a number of strategies for improving the interface between computers and older users have been identified. Some are based on technological adaptations, such as reducing mouse directional motion sensitivity and replacing double-clicking with easier commands. Other strategies include reducing the amount of text per page and increasing the type size of written material and web banners so they are large and easy to read (Glueckauf & Loomis, 2003).

Content can also be simplified to enhance older users' comprehension. For example, reducing "clutter" and keeping graphics simple can improve older adults' ability to master material presented on-line (Demiris, Finkelstein, & Speedie, 2001). Content can be simplified at the word, sentence, or text level (Singh, 2000). Other guidelines for increasing accessibility to health information for older adults or their caregivers can be found in books such as *Older Adults, Health Information and the World Wide Web* (Morrell, 2002b); *Aging, Communication, and Interface Design* (Laux, 2001), and *Human–Computer Interaction: Theory and Practice* (Jacko & Stephanidis, 2003).

Possible Negative Effects on Users

It also must be acknowledged that web-based interventions (like all other interventions) may exert potentially negative effects. Although the goal of a family involvement web site may be to provide information about dementia and possible coping strategies to improve caregiver adjustment and possibly resident quality of life, there are risks. For example, Proctor, Martin, and Hewison (2002) found that educating caregivers about dementia reduced caregiver depression but increased caregiver anxiety, primarily because of increased monitoring of the care recipient's symptoms. Similarly, although the coping strategies suggested on web sites targeting family caregivers of people with dementia are sometimes drawn from empirically validated interventions, there is no evidence that these strategies in isolation are effective for computer-based intervention participants or that strategies that have been shown to work for distressed caregivers will be effective for caregivers who are not distressed.

POTENTIAL CONTENT OF A
WEB-BASED FAMILY INVOLVEMENT INTERVENTION

Once initial planning is completed and the infrastructure is in place to implement a web-based family involvement intervention, the next step is to identify the services and content that can best meet the needs of families when delivering a web-based intervention protocol. Researchers have identified a number of empirically validated strategies to improve caregiver well-being and functioning (Gallagher Thompson et al., 2000). These strategies include providing information about symptoms of dementia, symptom management, stress management, latest research developments, and community resources. A planned web-based intervention can include any, or all, of these strategies.

A good example of a web-based version of such a program is Alzheimer's Caregiving Support Online, available at http://www.alz online.netindex.php (see the Resources section at the end of the chapter for more information on this web site and links to other useful sites). The state of Florida Department of Aging developed this particular web-based protocol. It is primarily an educational program about dementia, its treatment, and its consequences. Although it is still in the early stages of development, preliminary results have shown some positive effects on caregiver outcomes (Glueckauf & Loomis, 2003).

As stated earlier, some strengths of web-based interventions are their flexibility and their ability to meet the specific needs of their users. An example of a web-based intervention program and a method for assessing the intervention outcome is described in the following sections. The example is purposely ambitious to demonstrate the possibilities of a telehealth intervention, but even very simple interventions that incorporate single components of this program may prove successful and valuable for families of older adults with chronic disabilities living in nursing homes.

THE "EDUCATING FAMILIES AND IMPROVING COMMUNICATION" WEB-BASED INTERVENTION

The goal of this proposed intervention is to educate families about dementia and dementia care and to improve their communication with the residents, staff, and administration of the nursing home. Educational materials can focus on staff and family care responsibilities and problem solving with regard to dementia. The educational material is largely pedagogical and delivered through a series of web modules (see Table 10.1 for a list of potential modules). Everyone who logs on to the system is presented with the same information. For the pedagogical modules, users will log on and move through web-based lessons that present information on a variety of topics. Each module has a number of individual lessons on relevant topics that users can complete at their leisure.

Increasing communication requires interactive technology that will vary for each user. Interactive modules can include a variety of services. Interactivity can be kept to a minimum (e-mail or bulletin boards) or expanded to include "e-therapy" with social workers, psychologists, or other mental health professionals (King & Moreggi, 1998). The presence of more interactive web-based modules (see Table 10.2), such as bulletin boards, may enhance communication between family members and even staff and may create virtual support groups for important stakeholders.

Table 10.1 Modules to include in a computer-based family involvement intervention

Increasing caregiver knowledge and emotional well-being
    Basics of dementia
    Stress management
    Increasing positive emotion

Coping with challenging caregiving situations
    Understanding problem behaviors
    Managing problem behaviors
    Conflicts with other caregivers—staff
    Conflicts with other caregivers—family

What resources are available to me?
    Educational resources—links to federal, state, and community resources
    Legal resources—power of attorney, planning a living will
    Planning daily activities—How can I be involved?
    Communicating with care staff
    Communicating with nursing home management

Table 10.2.   Interactive modules

Communication—Providing easy e-mail access
   Between families and patients
   Between families and staff
   Between families and administration
   Between staff and administration
   Among staff
Videophone connection
   Between resident and family members
   Between health care professionals and family members
   Between family and staff members
Providing connections to on-line support groups
   Support groups for spouses
   Support groups for adult children
   Support groups for individuals with specific disorders
Calendar/daily activities
   General information
   Specific information

Technology can be simple, but, in some cases, more complicated strategies may also be effective if utilized properly. Complicated technology, such as a videophone, has been shown to be an effective approach to increasing communication. For example, family members who used videophones to stay in touch with elder relatives reported that the technology helped them feel more involved in the caring process (Savenstedt, Brunline, & Sandman, 2003). Videophone interactions with family members have the potential to increase the attentiveness of people with dementia and make them more focused on communicating (Savenstedt, Zingmark, & Sandman, 2003). Videophones have also been shown to increase the support provided by professional staff to informal caregivers (Magnusson et al., 1998). For some populations, an investment in videophone technology can be cost-effective, particularly if many family members live some distance away from a given nursing home and are unable to visit in person consistently.

On the other hand, simply providing e-mail access for residents who are cognitively able to use a computer can have positive results on psychosocial adjustment (White et al., 1999). Links to support groups can be provided in each of these e-mails. These groups, or Listservs, can be developed for families of a single nursing home or of multiple nursing homes. Links to national support groups for certain disorders could be included. Family members easily can get information about activities occurring for all of the residents in the nursing home, which may even prove more effective than other communication methods for some family members (e.g., those who are employed at full-time jobs and less likely to read mail carefully). Family members can use e-mails to keep up to date about the various activities available in the nursing home or to plan visits around activities, as well as to communicate with residents regarding their participation. It is also possible to post password-protected daily or weekly schedules for individual residents. Family members can use this information to assist in scheduling day-to-day activities for their relatives. This could be especially important for scheduling optional activities, such as visits to salons, that residents might enjoy but are unable to attend for whatever reason. Family members could also receive information about medical appointments and tests to help them monitor their relative's health more easily.

Assessing Outcomes

Good outcome research on the effectiveness of web-based interventions is scarce, so designers of web-based intervention protocols have an obligation to conduct outcome research (see Table 10.3). Assessment

Table 10.3.   Plan for assessing intervention outcome

Baseline measures
Alzheimer's Disease Knowledge Test
Nursing Home Resident Satisfaction Scale
Family Satisfaction Scale
Caregiving Distress Scale
Role Overload Scale
Loss of Intimate Exchange Scale
Computer Knowledge and Skill Survey
Intervention
Postintervention measures
Alzheimer's Disease Knowledge Test
Nursing Home Resident Satisfaction Scale
Family Satisfaction Scale
Caregiving Distress Scale
Role Overload Scale
Loss of Intimate Exchange Scale
Computer Knowledge and Skill Survey
Family Satisfaction with the Intervention

of effectiveness is relatively easy and can offer valuable information necessary to tailor interventions to the particular needs of nursing home residents, family members, and staff members across different facilities. Ideally, family members should be randomly assigned to an intervention or control group to truly assess the effectiveness of the intervention. Although this may not be possible in small nursing homes, outcome data still should be gathered. Before the intervention, family and resident satisfaction with care in the nursing home is assessed. Family members' perception of caregiving burden can also be assessed. Baseline data on family members' knowledge of dementia are gathered. Finally, data on family members' knowledge of and comfort with computers are collected. Because the intervention is computer based, it is possible that a lack of experience or comfort with computers could affect family satisfaction with the intervention. If many family members are uncomfortable with computers, a module on computers and the Internet may need to be added to the intervention.

Family members who are to receive the intervention should receive materials explaining the program and providing directions for using web programs. Prior to beginning the computer-based family involvement intervention, baseline measures of assessment should be conducted. Then, after a set time (probably 3–6 months), the assessment measures can be administered again to ascertain whether improvement has occurred. Several assessment measures to evaluate outcomes of the Educating Families and Improving Education intervention are described briefly in this section. Each of these measures is presented in the Appendix to the chapter.

Alzheimer's Disease Knowledge Test

Caregivers' knowledge about dementia can be assessed before and after the intervention with the Alzheimer's Disease Knowledge Test (Dieckman, Zarit, Zarit, & Gatz, 1988). This is a 20-item, multiple-choice questionnaire designed to assess knowledge about dementia.

Nursing Home Resident Satisfaction Scale

If residents are cognitively able, they should be asked about satisfaction with life in the nursing home. It is important to assess residents directly because family members and residents often disagree about the quality of care and accommodations provided in long-term care facilities (Gasquet, Dehe, Gaudebout, & Flissard, 2003). The Nursing Home Resident Satisfaction Scale (Zinn, Lavizzo-Mourey, & Taylor, 1993) is a brief 10-item scale that residents can complete relatively easily.

Family Satisfaction Scale

This scale is based on a statewide measure developed to assess family satisfaction with nursing home care in Ohio in 2003 (Ejaz, Straker, Fox, & Swami, 2003). It assesses satisfaction across 10 domains (Social Service and Communication, Direct Care and Nursing Assistants, Administration and Professional Nurses, Homelike and Spiritual Environment, Meals and Dining, Activities, Choice, Noise, Miscellaneous, and Overall Satisfaction). The Family Satisfaction Scale has good test–retest reliability.

Caregiving Distress Scale

The Caregiving Distress Scale is a 17-item scale that has five subscales (relationship distress, emotional burden, care-receiver demands, social impact, and personal cost) that assess the negative impact of caregiving on caregivers (Cousins, Davies, Turnbull, & Playfer, 2002).

Role Overload Scale

Role overload refers to feelings of exhaustion and fatigue resulting from caregiving demands. It is assessed with three items that are rated on a four-point scale (Pearlin, Mullan, Semple, & Skaff, 1990).

Loss of Intimate Exchange Scale

Loss of intimate exchange represents a caregiver's sense of loss of connectedness to the care recipient as a result of the progression of the care recipient's illness. It is measured with three items rated on a four-point scale (Pearlin et al., 1990).

Computer Knowledge and Skills Survey

This scale is based on scales used by Schumacher and Morahan-Martin (2001) to assess both computer knowledge and skills.

Family Satisfaction with the Intervention

This measure assesses many aspects of the intervention. Families are asked to report how comfortable they felt using the computer-based program and if they would recommend it to other family members. Families are also asked questions about the content of each module and if the information was valuable to them. Questions about the various services are included to determine if some options need to be revised or deleted. Finally, overall satisfaction with the intervention is assessed.

CONCLUSION

This chapter describes a possible intervention for family members of nursing home residents with dementia. The goal of the intervention is to educate families about dementia and dementia care and to improve communication between families, administrators, and staff members. The intervention combines static information and interactive services available through the World Wide Web to meet the needs of family members of residents. The proposed intervention is extensive. However, scaled-down (or expanded) versions are also feasible. If desired, similar interventions can be developed for administrators and staff. A possible method of outcome assessment is also described.

Helping families understand what roles they can potentially play in the lives of their relatives living in nursing homes can be beneficial in many ways. It may help reduce some of the dissatisfaction they experience with the care received in the nursing home. Educating families about daily care routines and why they are necessary may help them perceive the nursing home as less mechanistic. Families can learn about ways to stay involved with their relatives. Improved communication with staff may lead to more efficient or better care for residents. Technology can allow increased opportunities for interactions with residents, which can summarily boost residents' quality of life. Knowing more about dementia can help families make difficult decisions about their relatives' care. Overall, implementing a computer-based family intervention protocol can prove valuable for everyone involved—residents, family members, staff, and administrators.

REFERENCES

Adams, M.S., Oye, J., & Parker, T.S. (2003). Sexuality of older adults and the Internet: From sex education to cybersex. *Sexual and Relationship Therapy, 18*, 405–417.
Binstock, R.H., & Spector, W.D. (1997). Five priority areas for research in long-term care. *Health Services Research, 23*, 715–730.

Boise, L., & White, D. (2004). The family's role in person-centered care: Practice considerations. *Journal of Psychosocial Nursing and Mental Health Services, 42*(5), 12–20.

Britton, B.P. (2003). First home telehealth clinical guidelines: Developed by the American Telemedicine Association. *Home Healthcare Nurse, 21,* 703–706.

Buckwalter, K.C., Davis, L., Wakefield, B., Kienzle, M., & Murray, M. (2002). Telehealth for the elderly and their caregivers in rural communities. *Family and Community Health, 25,* 31–40.

Conover, L. (1997). The new generation of net surfers: Seniors. *Christian Science Monitor, 25,* 91.

Cousins, R., Davies, A.D.M., Turnbull, C.J., & Playfer, J.R. (2002). Assessing caregiving distress: A conceptual analysis and brief scale. *British Journal of Clinical Psychology, 41,* 387–403.

Crowe, B.L., Hailey, D.M., & Carter, R. (1992). Assessment of costs and benefits in the introduction of digital radiology systems. *Journal of Biomedical Computing, 30,* 17–25.

Davis, J.J. (2002). Disenfranchise the disabled: The inaccessibility of Internet-based health information. *Journal of Health Communication, 7,* 355–367.

Demiris, G., Finkelstein, S.M., & Speedie, S.M. (2001). Considerations for the design of a web-based clinical monitoring and educational system for elderly patients. *Journal of the American Medical Informatics Association, 8,* 468–472.

Dieckman, L., Zarit, S.H., Zarit, J.M., & Gatz, M. (1988). The Alzheimer's Disease Knowledge Test. *The Gerontologist, 28,* 402–408.

Duncan, M.T., & Morgan, D.L. (1994). Sharing the caring: Family caregivers' views of their relationship with nursing home staff. *The Gerontologist, 34,* 235–244.

Ejaz, F.K., Straker, J.K., Fox, K., & Swami, S. (2003). Developing a satisfaction survey for families of Ohio's nursing home residents. *The Gerontologist, 43,* 447–458.

Ferguson, E.W., Doarn, C.R., & Scott, J.C. (1995). Survey of global telemedicine. *Journal of Medical Systems, 19,* 35–46.

Finn, J. (1995). Computer-based self-help groups: A new resource to supplement support groups. *Social Work in Groups, 18,* 109–117.

Gallagher-Thompson, D., Lovett, S., Rose, J., McKibbin, C., Coon, D., Futterman, A., et al. (2000). Impact of psychoeducational interventions on distressed family caregivers. *Journal of Clinical Geropsychology, 6,* 91–110.

Gasquet, I., Dehe, S., Gaudebout, P., & Flissard, B. (2003). Regular visitors are not good substitutes for assessment of elderly patient satisfaction with nursing home care and services. *Journals of Gerontology. Series A, Biological Sciences and Medical Sciences, 58,* 1036–1041.

Glueckauf, R.L., & Loomis, J.S. (2003). Alzheimer's caregiver support online: Lessons learned, initial findings and future directions. *NeuroRehabilitation, 18,* 135–146.

Grau, L., Teresi, J., Burton, B., & Chandler, B. (1995). Family members' perception of the quality of nursing home care. *International Journal of Geriatric Psychiatry, 10,* 787–796.

Guilfoyle, C., Wootton, R., Hassall, S., Offer, J., Warren, M., Smith, D., et al. (2002). Videoconferencing facilities in providing care of elderly people. *Journal of Telemedicine and Telecare, 8*(Suppl. 3), 22–24.

Hailey, D., & Crowe, B. (2003). Assessing the economic impact of telemedicine. *Disease Management and Health Outcomes, 7,* 187–192.

Hailey, D., & Jennett, P. (2004). The need for economic evaluation of telemedicine to evolve: The experience in Alberta, Canada. *Telemedicine Journal and e-Health, 10,* 71–76.

Hendrix, C., & Sakauye, K.M. (2001). Teaching elderly individuals on computer use. *Journal of Gerontological Nursing, 27*(6), 47–53.

Herbert, L.E., Scherr, P.A., Bienias, J.L., Bennett, D.A., & Evans, D.A. (2003). Alzheimer disease in the U.S. population: Prevalence estimate by the 2000 census. *Archives of Neurology, 60,* 1119–1122.

Hertzberg, A., & Ekman, S.L. (2000). Views on the relationships and interactions between staff and relatives of older people permanently living in nursing homes. *Journal of Advanced Nursing, 31,* 614–622.

Hertzberg, A., Ekman, S.L., & Axelsson, K. (2003). "Relatives are resources, but . . . ": Registered nurses' views and experiences of relatives of residents in nursing homes. *Journal of Clinical Nursing, 12,* 431–441.

Hogue, E. (2003). Telehealth and risk management in home health. *Home Healthcare Nurse 21,* 699–701.

Irizarry, C., & Downing, A. (1997). Computers enhancing the lives of older people. *Australian Journal on Aging, 16,* 161–165.

Jacko, J., & Stephanidis, C. (2003). *Human-computer interaction: Theory and practice* (Part I). Mahwah, NJ: Lawrence Erlbaum.

Jennett, P., Yeo, M., Pauls, M., & Graham, J. (2003). Organizational readiness for telemedicine: Implications for success and failure. *Journal of Telemedicine and Telecare, 9,* 27–30.

Jerome, L.W., DeLeon, P.H., James, L.C., Folen, R., Earles, J., & Gedney, J.J. (2000). The coming age of telecommunications in psychological research and practice. *American Psychologist, 55,* 407–421.

Keats, S., Langdon, P., Clarkson, P.J., & Robinson, P. (2002). User models and user physical capability. *User Modeling and User-Adapted Interaction, 12,* 139–169.

Keefe, J., & Fancey, P. (2000). The care continues: Responsibility for elderly relatives before and after admission to a long term care facility. *Family Relations, 49,* 235–244.

King, S.A., & Moreggi, S. (1998). Internet therapy and self-help groups: The pros and cons. In J. Gackenback (Ed.), *Psychology and the Internet: Intrapersonal, interpersonal, and transpersonal issues* (pp. 77–109). San Diego: Academic Press.

Klein, B., & Richards, J.C. (2001). A brief Internet-based treatment for panic disorder. *Behavioral and Cognitive Psychotherapy, 29,* 113–117.

Kobb, R., Hilsen, P., & Ryan, P. (2003). Assessing technology needs for the elderly: Finding the perfect match for home. *Home Healthcare Nurse, 21,* 666–673.

Kolata, G. (2000). Web research transforms visit to the doctor. *New York Times,* March 6.

Koocher, G., & Morray, E. (2000). Regulation of telepsychology: A survey of state attorney generals. *Professional Psychology: Research and Practice, 31,* 503–508.

Kummervold, P.E., Gammon, D., Bergvik, S., Johnsen, J.A., Hasvold, T., & Rosenvingen, J. (2002). Social support in a wired world: Use of mental health discussion forums in Norway. *Nordic Journal of Psychiatry, 24,* 59–65.

Lange, A., van de Ven, J.P., Schrieken, B., & Emmelkamp, P. (2001). Interapy, treatment of post traumatic stress through the Internet: A controlled trial. *Journal of Behavior Therapy and Experimental Psychiatry, 32,* 73–90.

Laux, L.F. (2001). *Aging, communication, and interface design.* New York: Springer.

Liss, H.J., Glueckauf, R.L., & Ecklund-Johnson, E.P. (2002). Research on telehealth and chronic medical conditions: Critical review, key issues, and future directions. *Rehabilitation Psychology, 47,* 8–30.

Litwak, E., & Figuiera, J. (1970). Technological innovation and ideal forms of family structure in industrial society. In R. Hill & R. Konkig (Eds.), *Families in east and west: Socialization process and kinship ties* (pp. 348–396). Paris: Mouton.

Logue, R.M. (2003). Maintaining family connectedness in long-term care: An advanced approach to family centered nursing homes. *Journal of Gerontological Nursing, 20,* 24–31.

Maas, M.L., Reed, D., Park, M., Specht, J.P., Schutte, D., Kelley, L., et al. (2004). Outcomes of family involvement in care intervention for caregivers of individuals with dementia. *Nursing Research, 53,* 76–86.

Magnusson, L., Berthold, H., Chambers, M., Brito, L., Emery, D., & Daley, T. (1998). Using telematics with older people: The ACTION project. *Nursing Standard, 13*(5), 36–40.

Marquis, R., Freegard, H., & Hoogland, L. (2004). Influences on positive family involvement in aged care: An ethnographic view. *Contemporary Nursing, 16,* 178–186.

McAfee, D.F. (1999). Predictors of perceived emotional distress: Objective, subjective and demand burden, and health status of informal nursing home caregivers. *Dissertation Abstracts International Section A: The Humanities and Social Sciences, 59*(9-A), 3364.

McCrossin, R. (2003). Managing risk in telemedicine. *Journal of Telemedicine and Telecare, 9,* 36–39.

McIntosh, E., & Cairns, J. (1997). A framework for the economic evaluation of telemedicine. *Journal of Telemedicine and Telecare, 3,* 132–139.

McKay, H.G., Glascow, R.E., Feil, E.G., Boles, S.M., & Barrera, M.M. (2002). Internet based diabetes self-management and support: Initial outcomes from the Diabetes Network Project. *Rehabilitation Psychology, 47,* 31–48.

Morrell, R.W. (2002a). Older adults are getting online in the "Internet century." *Aging and Vision, 14,* 4–5.

Morrell, R.W. (2002b). *Older adults, health information and the World Wide Web.* Mahwah, NJ: Lawrence Erlbaum.

Murphy, K.M., Morris, S., Kiely, D.K., Morris, J.N., Belleville-Taylor, P., & Gwyther, L. (2000). Family involvement in special care units. *Research and Practice in Alzheimer's Disease, 4,* 229–239.

Normann, H.K., Asplund, K., & Norberg, A. (1998). Episodes of lucidity in people with severe dementia as narrated by formal carers. *Journal of Advanced Nursing, 28,* 1295–1300.

Pearlin, L.I., Mullan, J.T., Semple, S.J., & Skaff, M.M. (1990). Caregiving and the stress process: An overview of concepts and their measures. *The Gerontologist, 30,* 583–594.

Pillemer, K., Hegeman, C.R., Albright, B., & Henderson, C. (1998). Building bridges between families and nursing home staff: The Partners in Caregiving program. *The Gerontologist, 38,* 499–503.

Pillemer, K., Suitor, J.J., Henderson, C.R., Jr., Meador, R., Schultz, L., Robison, J., et al. (2003). A cooperative communication intervention for nursing home staff and family members of residents. *The Gerontologist, 43,* 96–106.

Proctor, R., Martin, C., & Hewison, J. (2002). When a little knowledge is a dangerous thing . . . : A study of carers' knowledge about dementia preferred coping style and psychological distress. *International Journal of Geriatric Psychiatry, 17,* 1133–1139.

Ritterband, L.M., Gonder-Frederick, L.A., Cox, D.J., Clifton, A.D., West, R.W., & Borowitz, S.M. (2003). Internet interventions: In review, in use and into the future. *Professional Psychology: Research and Practice, 5,* 527–534.

Rosen, J., Mittal, V., Muslant, B.H., Degenhgoltz, H., Castle, N., & Fox, D. (2003). Educating the families of nursing home residents: A pilot study using a computer based system. *Journal of the American Medical Directors Association, 3,* 128–134.

Ryan, A.A., & Scullion, H.F. (2000). Nursing home placement: An exploration of family carers. *Journal of Advanced Nursing, 32,* 1187–1195.

Sampson, J.P., Kolodinsky, R.W., & Greeno, B.P. (1997). Counseling and the information highway: Future possibilities and potential problems. *Journal of Counseling and Development, 75,* 203–212.

Savenstedt, S., Brunline, C., & Sandman, P.O. (2003). Family members' narrated experiences of communicating via video-phone with patient with dementia staying at a nursing home. *Journal of Telemedicine and Telecare, 9,* 216–220.

Savenstedt, S., Zingmark, K., & Sandman, P.O. (2003). Videophone communication with cognitively impaired elderly patients. *Journal of Telemedicine and Telecare, 9,* 52–54.

Scanlon, B. (2001). The future of the net: Surf's up for seniors. Retrieved October 31, 2004, from http://www.interactiveweek.com/articles

Schumacher, P., & Morahan-Martin, J. (2001). Gender, Internet and computer attitudes and experiences. *Computers in Human Behavior, 17,* 95–110.

Singh, S. (2000). Designing intelligence interfaces for users with memory and language limitation. *Aphasiology, 14,* 157–177.

Stevenson, J.G., Beck, C., Heacock, P., Mercer, S.O., O'Sullivan, P.S., Hoskins, J.A., Doan, J.R., & Schnell, J.F. (2000). A conceptual framework for achieving high quality care in nursing homes. *Journal of Healthcare Quarterly, 11,* 31–39.

Sussman, M.B. (1977). Family, bureaucracy, and the elderly individual: An organizational linkage perspective. In E. Shanas & M.D. Sussman (Eds.),

Family, bureaucracy, and the elderly (pp. 2–20). Durham, NC: Duke University Press.

Tate, D.F., Wing, R.R., & Winett, R.A. (2001). Using Internet technology to deliver a behavioral weight loss program. *JAMA, 285,* 1172–1177.

Trentin, G. (2004). E-learning and the third age. *Journal of Computer Assisted Learning, 20,* 21–23.

Weber, M. (1947). *The theory of social economic organization.* New York: Oxford University Press.

Weinberg, N., Uken, J.S., Schmale, J., & Adamek, M. (1995). Therapeutic factors: Their presence in a computer-mediated support group. *Social Work in Groups, 18,* 57–69.

White, H., McConnell, E., Clipp, E., Bynum, L., Teague, C., Navas, L., Craven, S., & Halbrecht, L. (1999). Surfing the net in late life. *Journal of Applied Gerontology, 18,* 358–378.

Winett, R.A., Roodman, A.A., Winett, S.G., Bajzek, W., Rovaniak, L.S., & Whitely, J.A. (1999). The effects of the Eat4Life Internet-based health behavior program on the nutrition and activity of high school girls. *Journal of Gender, Culture, and Health, 4,* 239–254.

Winker, M.A., Flanagin, A., Chi-Lum, B., White, J., Andrews, K., & Kennett, R.L. (2003). Guidelines for medical and health information sites on the Internet: Principles governing AMA web sites. *JAMA, 283,* 1600–1606.

Winzelberg, A. (1997). The analysis of an electronic support group for individuals with eating disorders. *Computers and Human Behavior, 13,* 393–407.

Zinn, J.S., Lavizzo-Mourey, R., & Taylor, L. (1993). Measuring satisfaction with care in the nursing home setting: The Nursing Home Resident Satisfaction Scale. *Journal of Applied Gerontology, 12,* 452–465.

RESOURCE

For further information or assistance in developing an Internet intervention, please contact

Valerie E. Tolbert, Ph.D.
Post-doctoral Research Fellow
Department of Behavioral Science, College of Medicine
The University of Kentucky
138 COMOB
Lexington, KY 40536-0086
E-mail: vetolb2@uky.edu
Telephone: 859-323-6028
Fax: 859-323-5350

On-line Resources

- A Place for Mom (http://www.aplaceformom.com)
  On this site, users can contact advisors through e-mail to help with

decision making on a variety of issues. Advisors can help connect users to resources and answer questions. This site can help users assess relatives' care needs and choose the appropriate level of care for those needs (assisted living, Alzheimer's disease care, nursing home, respite care, retirement communities, personal care, home care, and/or hospice care). The services are provided free of charge.

- Alzheimer's and Dementia Resources (http://www.therapeutic resources.com/alzheimers.html)
  This is a resource for health care professionals who work with people with dementia. It contains information about treatment strategies and treatment manuals, drug therapies, and other resources.

- Alzheimer's Caregiver Support Online (http://www.Alzonline.net/ index.php)
  This demonstration project is funded by the state of Florida. The site provides a variety of resources (reading rooms, expert forums, bulletin boards, chat rooms, Internet classrooms, and links to resources) for caregivers of individuals with Alzheimer's disease.

- American Psychological Association (http://www.apa/org/ethics)
  The American Psychological Association's Ethical Guidelines and Principles can be found here. There is information related directly to services provided by telephone, teleconferencing, and the Internet.

- American Telemedicine Association (http://www.atmeda.org)
  This web site was established in 1993. It has resources and information related to providers of telemedicine, including the *Home Telehealth Toolkit* and a state-by-state listing of legal issues related to telehealth services.

- HTML: An Interactive Tutorial for Beginners (http://www.dave site.com/webstation/html)
  Users can complete an interactive online tutorial on web page development at this site. Dave can teach users how to write HTML code, which is necessary for creating web pages.

- Dementia.com: Round-the-Clock Resources for Dementia (http:// www.dementia.com)
  This web site provides information about Alzheimer's disease and other dementias. It has medical information and tips on caregiving.

- Health Privacy and Policy Project (http://www.healthprivacy.org)
  This web site provided by the Health Privacy and Policy Project of

the Institute for Health Care Research and Policy at Georgetown University provides information on ways to protect patients' privacy.

- MedLinePlus: Trusted Health Information for You (http://www.nlm.nih.gov/medlineplus/nursinghomes.html)
This site provides information on a variety of topics related to nursing homes, including information on choosing a nursing home, alternatives to nursing homes, how to pay for care, and how to cope with family issues. It also provides relevant legal information, statistics, and links to other resources.

- Web Style Guide, Second Edition (http://www.webstyleguide.com)
This site provides basic information on developing a web site. It is a good place to begin to get an overview of the process.

10

Appendix

Alzheimer's Disease Knowledge Test

Nursing Home Resident Satisfaction Scale

Family Satisfaction Scale

Caregiver Distress Scale

Role Reversal Scale

Loss of Intimate Exchange Scale

Computer Knowledge and Skills Survey

Family Satisfaction with the Intervention

Alzheimer's Disease
Knowledge Test

For each question, circle the best answer among the choices provided.

1. The percentage of people over 65 who have severe dementia caused by Alzheimer's disease or a related disorder is estimated to be
    a. Fewer than 2%
    b. About 5%
    c. About 10%
    d. 20%–25%
    e. I don't know

2. The prevalence of Alzheimer's disease in the general population of the United States is expected to
    a. Decrease slightly
    b. Remain approximately the same
    c. Increase in proportion to the number of people over 65
    d. Nearly triple in the next 15 years
    e. I don't know

3. The cause of Alzheimer's disease is
    a. Old age
    b. Hardening of the arteries
    c. Senility
    d. Changes in the brain
    e. I don't know

Promoting Family Involvement in Long-Term Care Settings:
A Guide to Programs that Work, edited by Joseph E. Gaugler
© Copyright 2005 by Health Professions Press, Inc. All rights reserved.

4. Research in the role of heredity in Alzheimer's disease suggests that
   a. People with close relatives with Alzheimer's disease are at increased risk for developing Alzheimer's disease
   b. Alzheimer's disease is always transmitted genetically
   c. Alzheimer's disease is only inherited if both parents are carriers of the disease
   d. Alzheimer's disease is never inherited
   e. I don't know

5. Larger amounts of aluminum than normal have been found in the brains of some people with Alzheimer's disease. Studies on the role of aluminum in Alzheimer's disease
   a. Have determined it is a major cause
   b. Have established it plays a role in the onset of the disease
   c. Are inconclusive
   d. Have proven it is not a cause
   e. I don't know

6. A person suspected of having Alzheimer's disease should be evaluated as soon as possible because
   a. Prompt treatment of Alzheimer's disease may prevent more symptoms
   b. Prompt treatment of Alzheimer's disease may reverse symptoms completely
   c. It is important to rule out and treat reversible disorders
   d. It is best to institutionalize a person with Alzheimer's disease early in the course of the disease
   e. I don't know

7. Which of the following procedures is required to confirm that symptoms are due to Alzheimer's disease?
   a. Mental status testing
   b. Autopsy
   c. CT scan
   d. Blood test
   e. I don't know

8. Which of the following conditions sometimes resembles Alzheimer's disease?

    a. Depression

    b. Delirium

    c. Stroke

    d. All of the above

    e. I don't know

9. Which of the following is always present in Alzheimer's disease?

    a. Loss of memory

    b. Loss of memory, incontinence

    c. Loss of memory, incontinence, hallucinations

    d. None of the above

    e. I don't know

10. Although the rate of progression of Alzheimer's disease is variable, the average life expectancy after onset is

    a. 6 months to a year

    b. 1–5 years

    c. 6–12 years

    d. 15–20 years

    e. I don't know

11. Most research investigating lecithin as a treatment for Alzheimer's disease has concluded that it

    a. Reverses symptoms

    b. Prevents further decline

    c. Reverses symptoms and prevents further decline

    d. Has no effect on symptoms

    e. I don't know

12. Which of the following describes reactions Alzheimer's patients may have to their disease?

    a. They are unaware of the symptoms

    b. They are depressed

    c. They deny their symptoms

    d. All of the above

    e. I don't know

13. Sometimes patients with Alzheimer's disease wander from home. Caregivers can best manage this problem by

    a. Reasoning with the patient about the dangers of wandering

    b. Sharing feelings of concern with the patient in a calm and reassuring manner

    c. Making use of practical solutions, such as locking doors

    d. Remaining with the patient all of the time to prevent the behavior

    e. I don't know

14. Which is true about the treatment of patients with Alzheimer's disease who become depressed?

    a. It is usually useless to treat the depression because sadness and feelings of inadequacy are parts of the disease

    b. Treatments for depression may be effective in easing depressive symptoms

    c. Antidepressant medication should not be prescribed

    d. Proper medication can relieve depressive symptoms and prevent further intellectual decline

    e. I don't know

15. What is the role of nutrition in Alzheimer's disease?

    a. Proper nutrition can help prevent Alzheimer's disease

    b. Proper nutrition can reverse Alzheimer's disease

    c. Poor nutrition can make the symptoms of Alzheimer's disease worse

    d. Nutrition has no role in Alzheimer's disease

    e. I don't know

16. What is the effect of reminding people with Alzheimer's disease of the time and their location?

    a. It produces permanent gains in memory

    b. It slows down the course of the disease

    c. It increases confusion in 50% of patients

    d. It has no lasting effect on memory

    e. I don't know

17. People sometimes write notes to themselves as reminders. How effective is this for people with Alzheimer's disease?

    a. It can never be used because their comprehension is too limited

    b. It may be useful for a person with mild dementia

    c. It is a crutch that may contribute to further decline

    d. It may produce permanent gains in memory

    e. I don't know

18. When people with Alzheimer's disease begin having trouble performing self-care activities, many mental health professionals recommend that caregivers

    a. Allow the person to perform the activities regardless of the outcome

    b. Assist with the activities so the person can remain independent as long as possible

    c. Take over activities right away to prevent accidents

    d. Make plans to have the person moved to a nursing home

    e. I don't know

19. Medicare will pay for which of the following services for people with Alzheimer's disease?

    a. A physician's diagnostic evaluation of the person

    b. Nursing home care

    c. Home health care expenses

    d. All of the above

    e. I don't know

20. How many of the following are primary functions of the Alzheimer's Disease and Related Disorders Association (ADARA)?

    a. Conducting research

    b. Providing medical advice

    c. Providing family support and education

    d. Providing day care for people with Alzheimer's disease

    e. I don't know

Answers to quiz:

1–b; 2–c; 3–d; 4–a; 5–c; 6–a and c; 7–b; 8–d; 9–a; 10–c; 11–d; 12–d; 13–c; 14–b; 15–c; 16–b; 17–b; 18–b; 19–d; 20–a, b, c, and d

Nursing Home Resident Satisfaction Scale

Please help us to improve our services. Let us know our strengths and weaknesses. Using a scale from 1 (not so good) to 4 (very good), including N/A (not applicable), please rate your stay here on the following questions. Feel free to make any comments or suggestions.

1	2	3	4	5
not so good	okay	good	very good	N/A

Physician Services

1. How well do the doctors treat you? _____

2. How quickly do the doctors come when you ask to see them? _____

3. How would you rate your confidence in your doctors' abilities? _____

Nursing Services

4. How well do the nurses treat you? _____

5. How quickly do the nurses come when you ask to see them? _____

6. How would you rate your confidence in the nurses' abilities? _____

Other Services

7. How would you rate mealtime? (presentation, service, choices, taste) _____

8. How would you rate your room? (cleanliness, roommate, space, temperature) _____

9. How would you rate the amount of quiet and privacy? _____

10. How would you rate the daily schedule?
    (visitation, mealtime, bedtime, wake-up time)   _____

General Services
11. Considering everything, how would you
    rate your overall satisfaction? (doctor,
    nursing care facilities, and so forth)   _____

From Zinn, J.S., Lavizzo-Mourey, R., & Taylor, L. (1993). Measuring satisfaction with care in the nursing home setting: The Nursing Home Resident Satisfaction Scale. *Journal of Applied Gerontology, 12,* 452–465. Reprinted by permission.

Family
Satisfaction Scale

Rate how much you agree with each statement on a scale from 0
(strongly disagree) to 4 (strongly agree).

0	1	2	3	4
strongly disagree	disagree	neutral	agree	strongly agree

1. The social worker(s) follow up and
    respond quickly to my concerns. _____

2. The social worker(s) treat me with respect. _____

3. The social worker(s) treat the resident with respect. _____

4. I am satisfied with the quality of the
    social worker(s) in the facility. _____

5. The telephone calls are processed
    in an efficient manner. _____

6. The receptionist is helpful and polite. _____

7. Enough staff members are available to
    help the resident when he or she needs
    it (e.g., getting dressed, getting things). _____

8. During the evening, there is a staff person
    available to help the resident if he or she
    needs it (e.g., getting a blanket, getting a drink,
    changing positions). _____

9. A staff person checks to see if the resident is
    comfortable (e.g., asks if he or she needs a blanket,
    needs a drink, or needs a change in positions). _____

10. The resident looks well groomed and cared for. _____

11. The nursing assistants are gentle when
    they take care of the resident. _____

12. The nursing assistants treat the
    resident with respect. _____

13. The nursing assistants care about
    the resident as a person. _____

14. I am satisfied with the nursing
    assistants who care for the resident. _____

15. The administrative staff is available
    to talk with me. _____

16. The administrative staff treats me with respect. _____

17. The administrative staff cares about
    the resident as a person. _____

18. I am satisfied with the administrative
    staff in the facility. _____

19. The RNs and LPNs respond to my requests. _____

20. I am satisfied with the quality of
    the RNs and LPNs in the facility. _____

21. I am satisfied with the spiritual
    activities in the facility. _____

22. I think the facility should be cleaner. _____

23. The facility seems homelike. _____

24. The resident's belongings are safe in the facility. _____

25. I have a private space to visit the resident.
    (I can find places to talk to the resident in private.) _____

26. There is a comfortable place(s)
    for residents to sit outdoors. _____

27. I am satisfied with the resident's room. _____

28. I am satisfied with the safety
    and security of the facility. _____

29. Food is served at the right temperature
    (cold foods are cold; hot foods are hot). _____

30. The resident gets the food he or she likes. _____

31. The resident gets enough to eat in the facility. _____

32. The resident thinks the food is tasty. _____

33. I am satisfied with the food in the facility. _____

34. The facility activities provide
    things the resident likes to do. _____

35. The residents have enough to do in the facility. _____

36. The activities staff treats the resident with respect. _____

37. The activities staff cares about
    the resident as a person. _____

38. The resident is satisfied with
    the activities in the facility. _____

39. I am satisfied with the activities in the facility. _____

40. The staff provides me with (adequate)
    information about the different services
    in the facility. _____

41. The staff informs me (gives me clear
    information) about the daily rate. _____

42. The staff informs me (provides me with adequate information) about any changes. _____

43. The staff answers (adequately addresses) my questions about how to pay for care (e.g., private pay, Medicare, Medicaid). _____

44. I am satisfied with the manner in which the admission of the resident was handled. _____

45. The noise in the resident's room bothers me. _____

46. The noise in the public areas bothers me. _____

47. The resident can go to bed when he or she likes. _____

48. The resident chooses what clothes to wear. _____

49. The resident can have belongings that make his or her room feel homelike. _____

50. The staff leaves the resident alone if he or she wants to do nothing. _____

51. The resident has the opportunity to do as much as he or she wants to do. _____

52. The physical or occupational therapist spends enough time with the resident. _____

53. The resident's clothes get lost in the laundry. _____

54. The resident's clothes get damaged in the laundry. _____

55. I get adequate information from the staff about the resident's medical condition. _____

56. I am satisfied with the medical care in the facility. _____

57. I would recommend this facility
to a family member or friend.   _____

58. Overall, I am satisfied with the quality
of care the resident gets in the facility.   _____

Caregiver Distress Scale

Specific aspects of family life are affected by the demands of caregiving. With respect to your current situation as caregiver for _____, please use the 5-point scale below to indicate whether you personally agree or disagree with the following statements.

0	1	2	3	4
strongly disagree	disagree	neutral	agree	strongly agree

1. I take part in organized activities less. _____

2. I visit my family/friends less. _____

3. I take part in other activities. _____

4. I feel frustrated with caring for _____. _____

5. My relationship with _____ depresses me. _____

6. I feel pressure between giving to _____ and giving to others in the family. _____

7. I feel that my own health has suffered because of _____. _____

8. My relationship with _____ is strained. _____

9. Caring for _____ has made me nervous. _____

10. I feel _____ can only depend on me. _____

11. I feel resentful toward _____. _____

12. I feel helpless in caring for _____. _____

13. My relationship with _____
    no longer gives me pleasure.   _____

14. _____ tries to manipulate me.   _____

15. I feel overwhelmed by caring for _____.   _____

16. _____ makes more requests
    than are necessary.   _____

17. I feel that my personal life
    has suffered because of _____.   _____

Role Reversal Scale

How much does each statement describe you?

3	2	1	0
Completely	**Quite a bit**	**Somewhat**	**Not at all**

1. I am exhausted when I go to bed at night. _____

2. I have more to do than I can handle. _____

3. I don't have time just for myself. _____

4. I work hard as a caregiver but
    never seem to make any progress. _____

Promoting Family Involvement in Long-Term Care Settings:
A Guide to Programs that Work, edited by Joseph E. Gaugler
© Copyright 2005 by Health Professions Press, Inc. All rights reserved.

Loss of Intimate Exchange Scale

How much have you personally lost the following?

	3 Completely	2 Quite a bit	1 Somewhat	0 Not at all	
1. Being able to confide in your relative					_____
2. The person whom you used to know					_____
3. Having someone who knew you really well					_____

Computer Knowledge and Skills Survey

Please rate how much you agree on a scale of 0 (strongly disagree) to 4 (strongly agree) with each of the following statements.

0	1	2	3	4
strongly disagree	disagree	neutral	agree	strongly agree

1. I know how to use a computer. _____

2. I know how to access the Internet. _____

3. I know how to use e-mail. _____

4. I have searched for health information on the Internet. _____

5. I have purchased items on-line. _____

6. I have played computer games. _____

7. I know how to use word-processing programs. _____

8. I know how to use spreadsheet programs. _____

9. I think computers are very useful to me. _____

10. I feel comfortable using computers. _____

Promoting Family Involvement in Long-Term Care Settings:
A Guide to Programs that Work, edited by Joseph E. Gaugler

Family Satisfaction
with the Intervention

Place a checkmark next to each statement that describes how you feel about this program.

1. I found the intervention to be helpful. _____

2. I think my participation has improved my satisfaction with the care my relative receives. _____

3. I think my participation has positively affected my relative. _____

4. I know more about what I can do to help my relative. _____

5. I do more with/for my relative now than I did before the intervention. _____

6. I know more about dementia. _____

7. I know more about dementia care. _____

8. I understand more about how nursing homes work. _____

9. My communication with the staff has improved. _____

10. My communication with the administration has improved. _____

11. My communication with my relative in the nursing home has improved. _____

12. My communication with other family members has improved. _____

13. I thought the web-based lessons were more useful than the interactive communication-based services. _____

14. I would recommend this intervention to other people. _____

15. I had trouble getting on-line. _____

16. I had trouble using the system. _____

17. I would prefer the information be provided in other ways.

18. My lack of computer experience made the intervention useless for me. _____

19. Technical difficulties made the intervention useless for me. _____

20. Overall, I am very satisfied by my experiences with this intervention. _____

11

Challenges and Solutions in Promoting Family Involvement in Nursing Homes

Looking Toward the Next Generation of Programs

JOSEPH E. GAUGLER

As we have seen throughout the excellent contributions in this book, a number of promising strategies already exist to integrate families effectively into residential long-term care. These diverse and wide-ranging interventions have all shared a similar goal: to allow caregiving families to remain effectively involved in the lives of their loved ones well after the admission decision. Despite the emergence of a number of programmatic approaches to help families adapt to the nursing home transition, no efforts to date have attempted to critically integrate existing findings and results from these innovative efforts.

The goals of this final chapter are to highlight some of the barriers and limitations of the various program types reviewed in this book, and to help practitioners and long-term care providers avoid and manage some of the challenges implicit in implementing a family intervention. Following this overview of the barriers and challenges of administering family-based interventions in nursing homes, a series of practice recommendations are put forward to guide the design, implementation, and evaluation of future interventions. Underlying these practice recommendations is a discussion of what successful interventions will look like, based on the pioneering work of many of the chapter contributors. As with the preceding contributions, it is anticipated that this chapter will serve as a key resource for researchers and practitioners interested in facilitating families' transition to the nursing home experience.

BARRIERS, CHALLENGES, AND SOLUTIONS IN THE DEVELOPMENT AND ADMINISTRATION OF FAMILY INVOLVEMENT INTERVENTIONS

Lack of Conceptual Guidance

As indicated earlier, there is a noticeable lack of strong conceptual guidance when either studying family involvement dynamics in nursing homes or implementing and evaluating interventions designed to enhance family involvement and improve outcomes on the part of residents, families, and staff. This is problematic because little is known about the *mechanisms* that lead family members to become involved in nursing homes in the first place (i.e., the roles that family members choose to fill following institutionalization, such as advocate, care provider, and confidante) or to engage in negative types of involvement that may adversely influence quality of care (e.g., family conflicts with staff). The conceptual model presented by Gaugler in Chapter 1 is a starting point to understanding how family involvement occurs in nursing homes; developing interventions that consider the context of caregiving prior to admission to a nursing home and how this may influence family involvement during the move to a nursing home and long after is needed. In this manner, intervention components will be better able to target the strengths and resources of each family, leading to more flexible models that can produce wide-ranging, diffuse benefits for multiple stakeholders involved in the care of older adults living in nursing homes.

Integrating Family Involvement into Quality-of-Care Improvement Efforts

Current state-of-the-art quality-of-care efforts tend to emphasize services provided within facilities and their improvement. Although such approaches and philosophies are needed, taking advantage of the psychosocial resources that families provide to older adults living in nursing homes may offer an important dimension to existing quality-of-care protocols. As several researchers have noted, changes in the philosophy of nursing homes are often needed when improving quality of care (see Chapter 4), thus reducing the "medicalized" environments of many nursing homes. Although many long-term care providers choose to promote and advertise their facilities as "homelike" or "just like family," efforts beyond family council meetings are not widespread enough to actually encourage families to participate in regular activities that foster greater, socioemotionally enriching contact with relatives in nursing homes.

Some analyses have focused on the potential for long-term care facilities to debunk the myth of the "total institution" and instead remain fully integrated in the community context (e.g., Rowles, Conco-telli, & High, 1996). For example, concepts have been developed to reflect the exchange of people and communication between the facility and the community (*institutional permeability*) as well as the social, historical, psychological, and economic integration of facilities within their environmental contexts (*community integration*). Implementing less restrictive visiting hours can assist in creating a long-term care facility "without walls." Facilitating internal and external social activity (either through formal activities or the creation of private spaces that residents can utilize) may help residents identify with their home and family members beyond facility walls, as well as create strong social bonds to their home and "family" within the facility. The creation of these blurred institutional boundaries through social activity can result in an acceptance of the ways residents' lives within the long-term care environment continue as a function of their lives outside of the facility. The family involvement interventions (FIIs) presented in this book are starting points that could lead to a reframing of the medicalized, institutional nursing home environment to one that is more family friendly. In this regard, quality-of-care efforts could be maximized via involvement of existing family care resources in each facility.

Participation

Another important barrier and challenge to the implementation of any FII appears to be ensuring appropriate participation of family members. Particularly in facilities that are in areas where families are not in close geographic proximity, it is likely that promoting family involvement is daunting. Moreover, a distinct challenge that may emerge is engaging families in ways that allow for constructive feedback but at the same time avoid confrontation or conflict that may lead to a widening chasm between family and staff expectations.

The points highlighted by Anderson (see Chapter 2) apply not only to family councils but also to the administration of FIIs as a whole.

Specifically, the following steps can be implemented to promote family participation:

- *Connect with family members and residents—share the idea and concept of the FII and enlist participants' support to recruit other family members.* Utilization of other family members as recruitment tools is likely to enhance participation to a much greater extent than if facility liaisons contact family members to ask for their participation. "Spreading the word" about the program does not have to be limited to participating family members; capitalizing on community organizations such as churches, extension agents, local Area Agencies on Aging (AAAs), or other organizations in which family members are likely to take part can enhance not only family participation but also the overall community integration of the facility.

- *Contact the long-term care ombudsman, who can serve as a powerful advocate and a good source of information regarding families' rights and the functioning of successful FIIs.* The local long-term care ombudsman or other representatives from the local AAA can assist in emphasizing the importance of family involvement in the facility by contacting some family members directly or even speaking at preorganized facility events. Moreover, creating a strong working relationship with the AAA can provide the facility with access to a number of other informational resources for family members, staff, and even residents that can lead to improvement in the quality of care and quality of life in a given nursing home.

- *Connect with family councils and programs in other facilities that can share their experiences and prevent having to "reinvent the wheel."* Although many of the programs described in this book presume implementation in a single facility, creating a family involvement network across other local facilities may prove very effective and innovative. Capitalizing on the expertise of other family and staff members could help to augment existing FIIs and potentially boost the variety and success of family-based activities. It should also be noted that there is no reason to limit FII implementation to nursing home settings; creating FIIs that span the long-term care continuum (e.g., from assisted living facilities to nursing homes) could help create a philosophy of family involvement in long-term care for a given community, which could ease and facilitate older adults' transitions across care facilities.

- *Meet with the facility administrator—gaining the cooperation of the facility administrator is an important step in organizing a family intervention.* As Anderson emphasizes in Chapter 2, administrators should be visible as the FII is developed and implemented at any given facility. In addition to more "administrative" tasks (e.g., encouraging cooperation of staff, affording the group adequate meeting space, ensuring that the concerns of the group are taken seriously), periodic participation in components of FIIs such as family council meetings, family support groups, or even family–staff partnership meetings is necessary. Creating a commitment to offering a homelike facility environment in which families feel comfortable is likely a key component of any successful FII (Caron et al., 1999).

Anderson provides a number of other strategies to enhance family members' participation in FIIs (see Chapter 2). Although these were originally presented to facilitate participation on family councils, they have relevance across all types of FIIs:

- Utilization of orientation packets, posters and flyers, mailing lists, telephone calls, e-mails, receptions, and family "peer" contacts. Some of the strategies highlighted by Anderson include placing flyers or notices on cars in parking lots outside of a facility several days before a scheduled intervention session, mention of the FII at regular teas or other facility gatherings, and advertising in local newspapers and other media outlets (such as a web page).

- Flexibility in scheduling of FIIs to accommodate the diverse schedules of families.

- Selection of goals that are unique and achievable, particularly in the context of FIIs that include delineation of family and staff care responsibilities or those tasked with changing the "culture" of a given facility.

Flexibility in Content and Delivery

For group-based approaches, such as the programs outlined in Chapters 2 and 5, there is a distinct need to formulate content according to the needs of families in each facility. According to Peak (see Chapter 5), implementation of family support protocols tended to include consistent topics such as medication management, financial issues, and staff interaction with residents. Content for the other sessions varied considerably, however, and a strength of the family support program was its ability to remain flexible and responsive to the needs of its members. Moreover, some of the topics covered in group sessions are likely best addressed by outside experts, such as psychiatrists. This may result in particular challenges for those facilities that do not have the funds to pay for the time of these experts; as Peak suggested, use of gift certificates as well as flexible scheduling to take advantage of those willing to volunteer time to the facility may help address such issues. Some facilities may actually have experts among families and friends of residents or staff in the community; this may be another method to encourage outside participation in FIIs as needed.

Encouraging Family–Staff Interactions

Although many of the solutions promoted by Nikzad in Chapter 3 to encourage family–staff interaction are more systemic in nature, efforts at both the facility and the individual levels to interact with families may help to create a more positive environment and one that is more conducive to formal FII approaches. As suggested by Nikzad, staff members should make it a priority to let family members know where they are during visits and to verbally express how important family visits are to the residents. Moreover, staff members could provide oral invitations to family members to attend activities or even FII sessions, if needed. An underlying theme of Chapter 3 is to assure that staff members communicate to family members about how they have been able to effectively interact with a resident with cognitive impairments, which may help to create a greater level of understanding and appreciation of the care roles of both staff and family members.

Attrition

As mentioned by Drew (see Chapter 4) and others, the nature of life in nursing homes may create difficulty for any FII because not only are staff required to participate in daily care activities but also mortality among residents may place additional strains on families, thus affecting how they interact with the facility. Many of the FIIs presented in this book focus on family involvement in relation to the daily operation and care provision of the facility, but this does not necessarily encompass the concerns of all families with relatives living in a nursing home. For those families who have relatives receiving end-of-life care or who are faced with the discharge of a relative to some other facility, there is a need for FIIs to provide sensitive support and resources to help families (as well as the staff) manage these transitions. This is clearly an area that requires greater refinement in future interventions, as described later in this chapter.

Administrative Support

As intimated earlier and discussed in the detailed description of the Family Involvement in Care (FIC) intervention in Chapter 8, a particular barrier to implementing interventions in institutional settings is that nursing home administrators and staff may be reluctant to "adopt the intervention as their own." In contrast, staff and facilities are more likely to approach the implementation of the FII as a favor to the clinicians and researchers. Clearly, even more beneficial results might be possible if the commitment of the nursing staff to the intervention is improved. One way to circumvent this problem is to incorporate registered nurses (RNs) into any FII because these staff members often provide direction and leadership to unlicensed care personnel. As Specht, Reed, and Maas reported, RNs had the most "family-friendly" scores of nursing home staff and appeared to serve as an ideal conduit to family members. Collaborating and incorporating the perspectives of RNs could prove effective in promoting the successful implementation of FIIs to unlicensed care staff.

Timing of Delivery

Another key challenge to the successful administration of FIIs is *when* such programs are delivered in the care trajectories of families. Putting FIIs in place that target families who have just admitted their relatives to a facility in addition to family members of longer term residents may prove particularly beneficial to families and staff. As reported by Specht and colleagues in Chapter 8, family members participating in the FIC program often had a number of concerns about staff and services but were reluctant to directly address these problems with staff members. It is possible that FIIs such as the family–staff care partnership approaches detailed by Specht and colleagues (see Chapter 8) and Robison and Pillemer (see Chapter 9) might exert the most expansive benefits if they are implemented prior to family members' settling into a pattern of deference when making decisions regarding resident care.

Choosing the Right Facilitator

Particularly in FIIs that involve group-based exercises, selecting the appropriate facilitator is key to ensuring the success of a particular program. As outlined in detail by Robison and Pillemer in Chapter 9, naming an internal (e.g., director of social services) or external facilitator has several advantages and disadvantages. For example, an internal facilitator will likely have a stronger working knowledge of the facility and its culture and may be better suited to identifying and working with different sectors of the nursing home to facilitate change if needed. Moreover, an internal facilitator can potentially offer stability following the initial stages of an FII and can move forward with recommendations proposed by participating family and staff members. Perhaps most important, an internal facilitator can save facilities money and resources when compared with bringing in an external facilitator. In contrast, an external facilitator may create more open channels of communication between participants in an FII because an external facilitator may be perceived as less likely to break bonds of confidentiality and inform administrators or others of group proceedings. As Robison and Pillemer emphasized, it is likely that most nursing homes will utilize in-house facilitators for group-based interventions (primarily social work staff), and, although the evaluations suggest that this is a useful approach, some flexibility is necessary to maximize the impact of group-based FII components. In particular, trying both internal and external facilitators separately at the outset of an FII may help facilities choose which approach is most appropriate.

Staff Training and Payment

Who should be trained to deliver FIIs, and how should staff be paid for participating in them? As Robison and Pillemer discussed in Chapter 9, these are challenging issues in the development and implementation of FIIs. To address the first question, the Partnership in Caring intervention trained both nurses and nursing assistants as a single group; this appeared effective not only in the implementation of the intervention but also in the overall facilitation of improved nurse–nursing assistant communication and working relationships. The training of nurses and nursing assistants could be broadened to include other staff members who work closely with families, such as social workers or possibly even activity directors. In terms of staff payment, Robison and Pillemer advise that staff receive their regular working wage during training phases of FIIs. In particular, staff members who receive lower hourly wages (e.g., nursing assistants) in all likelihood would depend on regular payment in order to participate in an FII. Paying staff for their participation also emphasizes the facility's commitment to improving family involvement and quality of life in the nursing home; incorporating FII training into regular in-service education may embed the philosophy of family outreach and involvement into the overall facility culture.

Manualized Intervention Materials

Although many of the FIIs described in this book have supporting materials to guide the implementation and delivery of the intervention (see the end of each chapter for contact and resource information), some of the components of the FIIs, particularly those that are more exploratory (e.g., computer-based FIIs; see Chapter 10) may have few supporting materials to guide interested staff in implementing a newly developed FII. This can be a concern because preparation is key to administering an effective multicomponent FII (see Chapter 9). For example, in the Family Visit Education Program (FVEP) outlined by Dr. McCallion in Chapter 6, the FII manual, or "protocol," includes a leader manual, a family participant workbook that provides reviews of FVEP materials and assignments, and a "train-the-trainer" videotape that outlines each of the key components of the FVEP. Although it is recommended that interested practitioners who wish to implement FIIs in their given facilities take advantage of developed manuals and resources, these may not be fully available or developed; moreover, if facilities wish to implement certain components of an FII or develop their own FII, it is important to develop training protocols that meet the needs of each facility. This book is a first step in providing a resource to facilities to develop and promote effective family involvement, but it is also recognized that the needs of facilities as well as the nascent nature of research in this area require innovation on the part of service providers. The more programs are manualized and documented, the more likely these new-generation FIIs can be subject to evaluation.

Professional Background of FII Facilitators

Another challenge that may influence the successful implementation
of an FII is the educational and professional experience of a group
moderator, if that is what the FII requires. For example, in the FVEP
(see Chapter 6), a practitioner with a master's degree who also had
experience working with residents with cognitive impairments and
their family members administered the program. Although some facilities may have staff on site with similar credentials (e.g., a director of
social services with a master's degree in social work), other facilities
may have difficulty freeing staff time and resources to commit such an
individual to the administration of an FII. When coupled with the
preparation and training necessary to effectively implement an FII such
as the FVEP (see Chapter 6), facilities may be reluctant to commit
highly trained staff to an FII. Again, however, it should be noted that
if the FII to be delivered has extensively documented training materials
(such as the FVEP), the need for a master's-level practitioner or similar
type of staff person to deliver an FII may be mitigated; a junior-level
social worker or other staff member may be just as well suited to deliver
a multicomponent intervention such as the FVEP, given the time to
review the materials and gain mastery over its delivery.

Confidentiality and Participation in an FII

With increasing concerns regarding resident confidentiality and privacy, a key issue to be addressed prior to and during the administration
of an FII is how to remain sensitive to these concerns, particularly in
FIIs in which revealing information may be provided about a resident
(e.g., see Chapter 7). As discussed by Hepburn and Caron in their
presentation of the Family Stories Workshop, some family members
were concerned about their responsibility toward their relatives when
presenting stories and narratives. Some participants in the Family Stories Workshop even wondered whether informed consent was needed
from the resident (a problematic issue because the Family Stories Workshop is designed for residents who have dementia). Hepburn and Caron
suggested that these concerns be addressed by emphasizing to participants that they act as *surrogate* storytellers when creating the story of
their relatives' lives and that poetic license is also appropriate in the
context of the Family Stories Workshop. Moreover, facilities are
encouraged not to be cowed by privacy or confidentiality concerns

when implementing such innovative and clearly beneficial programs as the Family Stories Workshop. Such concerns can be resolved with, for example, simple verbal assent procedures, incorporating or even including residents in the development of the narrative with family members, and emphasizing that the information derived from FIIs such as the Family Stories Workshop is presented directly in the facility (much as health-related information is) to improve quality of life and quality of care in the nursing home.

Enhancing Staff Participation in FIIs When It Is Needed

As Hepburn and Caron (see Chapter 7) and others have noted in their presentation of FIIs, the success for any of these programs largely relies on the facility "culture," or the facility's willingness to be creative and promote family involvement with innovative methods (and such sentiment more often than not emanates from the administrator). As Hepburn and Caron as well as Specht et al. (see Chapter 8) emphasize, the level of administrative commitment to and enthusiasm for the given FII by the facility, administrators, and often senior nursing staff appears to be the principal determinant of staff participation in FIIs and the overall effectiveness of these programs. In the instances provided in this book, large groups of staff were enthusiastic about and available to participate in various FIIs. In other cases, many staff members did not participate, often because facilities were unable or unwilling to free up staff time for participation. In the Family Stories Workshop, one solution was videotaping the presentations and making these tapes available to facilities so that staff members who were unable to participate could do so to some extent; however, such an approach may not be feasible for those FIIs that rely on direct family–staff role partnerships and care plans (e.g., see Chapter 8).

Unfortunately, there are no easy or readily available answers in instances in which facilities are unwilling to participate in FIIs because such barriers are due as much to the institutional and routinized environment of nursing homes as they are to personal characteristics of a particular administrator or staff person. The best that interested practitioners can do is to incorporate less intensive and more flexible FII components that can be easily integrated into the nursing home and work with not only individuals inside the facility but also those outside (e.g., corporate management, long-term care ombudsmen) to create a more family-friendly culture at a resistant facility.

PRACTICE RECOMMENDATIONS

Multicomponent Approaches

Research on psychosocial interventions for family caregivers in the community consistently concludes that multifaceted programs that provide individualized services are more effective than most commonly designed caregiver interventions that emphasize only education and support (Schulz et al., 2002). The FIIs summarized in the book build on these prior findings by further emphasizing the need for multicomponent approaches when enhancing family adaptation and involvement following the admission of an elderly relative to a long-term care facility. As the programs summarized by Specht et al. (see Chapter 8) and Robison and Pillemer (see Chapter 9) suggest, strategies that combine support with more individually tailored components (e.g., staff meetings with individual family members to formulate care plans) represent the state of the art in family-based intervention in long-term care. Further identification of components that are useful when intervening on behalf of families will continue to refine the trend toward multicomponent strategies. Such research will also help to highlight the need for interventions that are flexible and tailored to the diverse needs of caregiving families.

Several conceptual tools are available to practitioners that can guide the development of more complex, multicomponent intervention approaches, such as family life education (FLE) principles. The main goal of FLE is to strengthen and enrich individuals and family well-being (e.g., Arcus, 1992; Brubaker & Roberto, 1992). Family-based intervention strategies within the FLE framework could emphasize the following:

1. The quality and continuity of family relationships prior to, during, and after placement

2. Understanding how individuals and families have managed stressful situations in the past when developing strategies to improve family adaptation to the residential care experience

3. The implementation of approaches that involve multiple family members across generations who are likely to visit and remain integrated in the resident's life, such as grandchildren

4. Reliance on families and residents themselves as information resources to guide individualized care plans

5. The recognition that variations in gender, kin relationship, and racial/ethnic background demand flexible programs in contrast to the "one intervention fits all" approach

Multicomponent family-based programs in long-term care that incorporate FLE guidelines may prove even more effective than past interventions for facilities, staff, families, and residents.

Timing

There is a paucity of approaches that alleviate the potential upheaval that may affect families during and immediately after admission of an older relative to a nursing home. Locating a suitable nursing home, notifying and preparing the care recipient for the transition, and coping with the subsequent emotional issues often place significant stress on the entire family. Unfortunately, practical interventions and support programs are often inadequate or nonexistent, leaving families to navigate the long-term care system without the support and assistance of a trained professional (Dellasega & Mastrian, 1995; Ryan & Scullion, 2000). Although some existing interventions to promote family involvement following admission may help address the needs of families of newly admitted residents (e.g., see Chapter 5), there is a clear gap in service availability for family members just beginning to manage the ramifications of nursing home admission. Evaluations of strategies designed to assist family members of newly admitted residents would provide a clearer contribution to the literature and serve as an integrative scientific bridge with family-based interventions oriented to improve family involvement and family–staff relationships for "long-stay" residents.

Incorporation of Multiple Stakeholder Perspectives

Programs that appear to exert the greatest impact consider multiple stakeholders when attempting to increase and facilitate family involvement. For example, interventions that incorporate family and staff in collaborative partnerships/contracts have reported efficacy in improving family involvement in some areas (e.g., Anderson, Hobson,

Steiner, & Rodel, 1992; see also Chapters 6, 8, and 9). In addition to assessing the benefits of these programs for family–staff relationships, these interventions could measure potential outcomes for residents and the facility environment more consistently in order to document the overall ramifications of family-based intervention programs. In particular, it appears that the success of FIIs depends on the culture of each facility (e.g., Caron et al., 1999). It is likely that the divergent or convergent views of social workers, families, residents, and staff members may influence the overall effectiveness of a given intervention, and practitioners must take steps to ensure that programs are flexible enough to develop services and activities that address the complex interrelationships between these key individuals. To date, little is known about whether the overall goals of particular interventions mesh with those of important stakeholders. Future evaluations that document the interactive relationship between program implementation and facility environment/culture over time and how various stakeholders disagree or work together would help practitioners determine which approaches are most feasible in their respective facilities.

Considering the Transitions of Families from Care Provision to Discharge/Bereavement

Although many existing FIIs cast a relatively wide net to increase participation, the content of many programs may be skewed to those family members with long-stay relatives in nursing homes. Incorporating family perspectives into the culture of the facility is important, and the valiant efforts made by existing FIIs to do so are praiseworthy, but more comprehensive and integrated family programs may be necessary to meet the diverse needs of families. Specifically, as much of the research on family caregiving has acknowledged, caregiving is often a career that can last many years (particularly in the case of chronic diseases such as dementia) and encompasses many transitions, such as onset into caregiving responsibilities, bereavement, and, pertinent to this book, admission to a long-term care facility. Existing research and, to some extent, clinical practice have failed to acknowledge that family care often does not abate following admission, and many families remain involved in the lives of their relatives at admission and for many years thereafter. For these reasons, FIIs should be tailored to take the caregiving career into account; as opposed to programs that are primarily geared to families who already have relatives in a nursing home, more dynamic and integrated approaches are needed that include components to help families deal with

1. Initial orientation to the facility, its operation, its environment, and its management of financial, care, and personal issues

2. How residents are cared for in acute rehabilitative settings as well as more long-term, skilled care settings

3. How to find information and resources both within and outside of the facility, such as the ombudsman, other community-based or residential long-term care resources, and local AAAs

4. How to manage and deal with increased dependence or worsening health of their relative that may lead to discharge

5. How to navigate hospice services and cope with bereavement

Although these are just preliminary components of an FII that attempt to meet the needs of families *over time*, it appears, from what is now available, that families may need the most flexible type of FII possible to help address the changing needs of the relative, both at admission and for some time afterward. Augmenting information components such as those listed here with the more collaborative, group-based activities of staff–caregiver partnerships, Family Stories Workshops, or family support groups may prove particularly appealing to families with relatives in nursing homes who must manage the many health-related transitions that can occur in their relative's care.

Establishing Relationships Outside of the Facility

Another theme that seems to underpin the most successful FIIs is their ability to maintain strong working relationships with organizations and individuals outside of their nursing home. This may be key to facilitating the proper type of environment that is integrated within the community and, as a result, becomes more open to facilitating family involvement and other cooperative agreements with individuals outside of the nursing home. For example, some research has focused on the potential for long-term care facilities to debunk the myth of the "total institution" and instead remain fully integrated in the community context (e.g., Rowles et al., 1996; see earlier discussion). Research currently underway (e.g., see http://www.mc.uky.edu/Permeability) is directly examining how quality of life in residential long-term care settings such as nursing homes can be promoted via strong, positive relationships between residents, staff, and family members and others outside of the facility (i.e., permeability; see Figure 11.1). It is likely that this dynamic plays an important role in the success of FIIs; those facilities that are more institutional and closed off from their surrounding communities will have a more difficult time implementing FIIs (although it is likely these are the types of nursing homes where they are most needed) because these nursing homes may have a more difficult time seeing the necessity of creating strong bonds and working relationships with people and organizations outside of the facility. However, current research will strongly suggest that such steps are necessary to create the type of facility culture that can effectively support and maintain family involvement.

A potential starting point when developing FIIs to capitalize on the community outside of the facility is to invite outside facilitators to administer group-based intervention activities (see Chapter 9). Some examples are local social workers or even former employees of the nursing home (e.g., a social worker) who would have some interest in remaining involved in the nursing home on a part-time basis. In many ways, this could serve as an ideal arrangement because such an individual, while bringing an outside, community perspective, would also have some working knowledge of the culture of the nursing home. Other possibilities include inviting representatives from community organizations such as Cooperative Extension offices or even collaborating and sharing staff with other residential care facilities in the area and region. Taking these steps to move beyond the traditional facility walls and integrate the nursing home in the surrounding community is likely to broaden its appeal not only to families but also to a number of other key stakeholders.

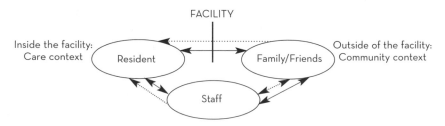

Figure 11.1. Theoretical model of institutional permeability. (Key: ——————, socioemotional exchange; ...., instrumental exchange.)

Booster Sessions

For those programs with long-term goals and outcomes, there is a distinct need to incorporate "booster sessions," or intervention components that are delivered after the initiation of the FII to ensure maintenance of intervention benefits. As Robison and Pillemer indicated in their evaluation of the Partnership in Caring program (see Chapter 9), the strongest effects of the FII were found at the first posttest assessment, and effects appeared to attenuate after 6 months and beyond. Somewhat similar findings were evident in the FIC intervention summarized by Specht and colleagues (see Chapter 8). These findings point to the diminishing impact of some FIIs over time, due in part to the need to reinforce or reestablish the skills conferred in the initial stages of the FII. Booster sessions can occur some time after the initial implementation of an FII and can also be shorter (or, more "streamlined") than full program components. In addition to maintaining the effectiveness of a given FII, booster components are likely to be less time consuming than the initial stages of the program and could continue the overall benefits of an FII for longer periods of time.

Creating Frontline and Intensive FIIs

Although many of the FIIs presented in this book have demonstrated notable success in improving family involvement and staff–family relationships, they also require considerable investment on the part of facilities, staff, and family members. Family–staff partnerships and group-based perspectives in particular are more time-intensive intervention strategies that may have difficulty meeting the needs of families who have busy schedules or possibly do not even live near the nursing home. In these instances, developing more frontline intervention protocols that are more flexible in working with the time demands of families and staff may be initially effective in guiding families into more complex intervention components. For example, utilizing Internet-based or CD-ROM materials to introduce families to the nursing home and its culture and staff, creating e-mail lists or even web-based discussion boards to offer virtual support and interaction, and developing Internet-based resources that can capitalize on the large amount of advocacy and information materials related to long-term care (e.g., the Nursing Home Compare site maintained by the Centers for Medicare and Medicaid Services; see http://www.medicare.gov, and click on

"Compare Nursing Homes in Your Area") would create cost-effective approaches that can enhance how families remain involved in nursing homes. Following these initial efforts, family members could be identified to participate in more time-intensive intervention modules to directly address staff–family relationships or other issues. In this manner, cost-effectiveness and the overall efficacy of future FIIs could be improved significantly. Tolbert and Basham provided a number of "virtual" resources and strategies that could serve as important frontline FIIs that may later transition into face-to-face, group-based, and individualized program components (see Chapter 10).

Finding the Voice of the Resident

Noticeably absent in the research literature and even in the evaluation of many of the FIIs mentioned in this book is the perspective of residents themselves. Although several of the FIIs are oriented to facilitate family involvement when the resident has severe cognitive impairment, it is still problematic that many of the most refined FIIs seem to focus on family–staff relationships and avoid the dynamic of family–resident or resident–staff relationships. Some of the work on family involvement, institutional permeability, and quality of life in long-term care strongly emphasizes the consideration of family, staff, and resident perspectives in concert (e.g., Gaugler, 2005; Gaugler, Anderson, & Leach, 2003; Gaugler, Leach, & Anderson, 2004). For example, considering family–staff, family–resident, and staff–resident relationships and social exchanges within an FII would be integral to developing an intervention that can positively influence a wide array of outcomes not only for families but for staff and residents as well (e.g., see Figure 11.1). This manifestation of the facility–staff–family–resident dynamic could be key to intervening and improving outcomes in nursing homes.

Similarly, measurement from the resident's perspective has been notably lacking. Current statistics suggest that 50%–75% of nursing home residents have some type of dementia (Magaziner et al., 2000). It is generally assumed that researchers would therefore have a difficult, if not impossible, time administering open-ended or closed-ended measures that collect reliable information on key resident outcome measures, such as quality of life. Because of such cognitive difficulties, there has been some reluctance among researchers and practitioners to assess quality of life or other dimensions on the part of residents. However, an increasing number of studies are recognizing that individuals with dementia, even those in more severe stages of the condition, can provide reliable information on their mood and quality of life (Brod, Stewart, Sands, & Walton, 1999; Kane et al., 2003; Lawton, van Haitsma, & Klapper, 1996; Logsdon, Gibbons, McCurry, & Teri, 1999). These methods could be adapted and included in future evaluations to more effectively discern the role of family-based interventions in improving resident outcomes. Moreover, practitioners and researchers alike, when building or refining FIIs for their needs, are encouraged to incorporate resident perspectives because it is likely that family involvement is only one component in actually creating long-term care environments that are socially and psychologically enriching.

CONCLUSION

Family caregiving for older adults with disabilities is in many respects a career, with the admission of the relative to a long-term care facility a key transition. As interventions have emerged to promote family involvement and improve family–staff relationships in residential long-term care, a number of important issues remain in the literature. Future FIIs that recognize the complexity and diversity of the family care context will refine current strategies to assist families. In addition, programs that have multiple components and consider a variety of stakeholder perspectives will help facilitate the widespread implementation of effective programs. In this manner, family-based interventions will achieve increased levels of success following the transition to residential care and will lead to the overarching goal that families, residents, care providers, researchers, and policy makers share: to create the best possible quality of life in nursing homes.

REFERENCES

Anderson, K.H., Hobson, A., Steiner, P., & Rodel, B. (1992). Patients with dementia: Involving families to maximize nursing care. *Journal of Gerontological Nursing, 18*, 19–25.

Arcus, M.E. (1992). Family life education: Toward the 21st century. *Family Relations, 41*, 390–393.

Brod, M., Stewart, A.L., Sands, L., & Walton, P. (1999). Conceptualization and measurement of quality of life in dementia: The Dementia Quality of Life instrument (DQoL). *The Gerontologist, 39*, 25–35.

Brubaker, T.H., & Roberto, K.A. (1992). Family life education for the later years. *Family Relations, 42,* 212–221.

Caron, W., Hepburn, K., Luptak, M., Grant, L., Ostwald, S., & Keenan, J. (1999). Expanding the discourse of care: Family constructed biographies of nursing home residents. *Families, Systems, & Health, 17,* 323–335.

Dellasega, C., & Mastrian, K. (1995). The process and consequences of institutionalizing an elder. *Western Journal of Nursing Research, 17,* 123–140.

Gaugler, J.E. (2005). Staff–resident relationships across the long-term care landscape. *Journal of Advanced Nursing, 49,* 377–386.

Gaugler, J.E., Anderson, K.A., & Leach, C.R. (2003). Predictors of family involvement in residential long-term care. *Journal of Gerontological Social Work, 42,* 3–26.

Gaugler, J.E., Leach, C.R., & Anderson, K.A. (2004). Correlates of resident psychosocial status in long-term care. *International Journal of Geriatric Psychiatry, 19,* 773–780.

Kane, R.A., Kling, K.C., Bershansky, B., Kane, R.L., Giles, K., Degenholtz, H.B., et al. (2003). Quality of life measures for nursing home residents. *Journals of Gerontology. Series A, Biological Sciences and Medical Sciences, 58,* M240–M248.

Lawton, M.P., van Haitsma, K., & Klapper, J. (1996). Observed affect in nursing home residents with Alzheimer's disease. *Journals of Gerontology. Series B, Psychological Sciences and Social Sciences, 51,* P3–P14.

Logsdon, R.G., Gibbons, L.E., McCurry, S.M., & Teri, L. (1999). Quality of life in Alzheimer's disease: Patient and caregiver reports. *Journal of Mental Health and Aging, 5*(1), 21–32.

Magaziner, J., German, P., Zimmerman, S.I., Hebel, J.R., Burton, L., Gruber-Baldini, A.L., et al. (2000). The prevalence of dementia in a statewide sample of new nursing home admissions age 65 and over: Diagnosis by expert panel. *The Gerontologist, 40,* 663–672.

Rowles, G.D., Concotelli, J.A., & High, D.M. (1996). Community integration of a rural nursing home. *Journal of Applied Gerontology, 15,* 188–201.

Ryan, A.A., & Scullion, H.F. (2000). Nursing home placement: An exploration of the experiences of family caregivers. *Journal of Advanced Nursing, 32,* 1187–1195.

Schulz, R., O'Brien, A., Czaja, S., Ory, M., Norris, R., Martire, L.M., et al. (2002). Dementia caregiver intervention research: In search of clinical significance. *The Gerontologist, 42,* 589–602.

RESOURCES

Please see Chapter 1 for information about Dr. Gaugler's research and for publication information. If you have comments, questions, or concerns about the resources and programs presented in this book and how to implement a family involvement intervention in your facility, please contact

Joseph E. Gaugler, Ph.D.
Assistant Professor
School of Nursing
The University of Minnesota
6-150 Weaver-Densford Hall, 1331
308 Harvard Street S.E.
Minneapolis, MN 55455
E-mail: gaug0015@umn.edu
Phone: 612-626-2485
Fax: 612-626-2359

Index

Page numbers followed by *t* or *f* indicate tables or figures, respectively.